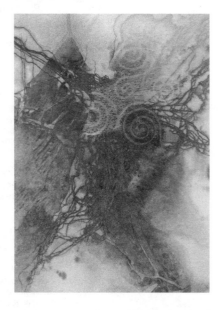

W*ise Warrior* came to life in the summer of 2002. Using a mixed media of watercolor, colored pencil and torn paper, Linda Gerard Dzik created a female image that stands in a strong and solid yoga warrior pose. *"As a watercolorist, when I create an abstract, I let the paint determine the illustration. I decided to experiment with a special textured paper and I glued it into wet paint. After it dried, a breast was obvious, a woman emerged and the Wise Warrior was born."* Linda had considered donating the picture to a benefit auction shortly afterward, but her husband intuitively suggested that Wise Warrior had another purpose. It hung in Linda's studio for nearly two years until we met in July of 2004. We agreed that its destiny was the cover of The Blue Tattoo Club. The illustration is rich with symbolism for all women, particularly breast cancer survivors. Some see wings. Some see a third eye. Some see the spiral of life in the breast area. It speaks to each person differently. We see a strong, solid woman poised and ready to take on whatever may come her way.

ISBN: 0-9763081-7-7
Library of Congress Control Number:
2004097792

Printed in the United States of America

www.bluetattooclub.com

Special thanks to:

Songs for the Inner Child
by Shaina Noll
©Singing Heart Productions
7 Avenida Vista Grande #244
Santa Fe, NM 87508
505/466-2886
www.shainanoll.com
All rights reserved.

How Could Anyone
Words and music by Libby Roderick
©Libby Roderick Music 1988
Turtle Island Records
P.O. Box 203294
Anchorage AK 99520
907/278-6817 libbyr@alaska.net
www.alaska.net/~libbyr/
All rights reserved.

Always Remember
by Roy Lessin
©DaySpring Cards, Inc.
Used by permission.
www.dayspring.com

Rob Hagen, the photographer who tramped through the woods
with us to find the perfect setting for our group photo.

Jerry Armstrong of J.B. Kenehan, Inc. for his interest in and support of our first publication.

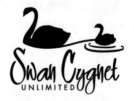

www.swancygnet.com

*This book is dedicated to Jenell Olson,
my creative muse, my winsome sage,
my unforgettable friend.*

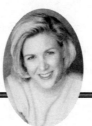

Delbert & Loretta,
You are both very the
special friends over the
years to the smiles.

Christy

What is the Blue Tattoo Club?

*A*nyone who has ever undergone radiation treatment for breast cancer will know the source of this book's title. For the fortunately uninitiated, The Blue Tattoo Club refers to the blue tattoos inscribed on women's chests that mark forever the area toward which the radiation beams are directed.

This book is a collection of the real and relevant experiences of women who have encountered breast cancer in their lives. It is a book for all women: whether they are waiting for test results; have just been diagnosed; are in the midst of treatment; have completed their own journey or care about another woman at any of these stages.

The twelve women who express themselves here recall their own hopes and heartaches as they made their individual choices regarding treatment. At the time of diagnosis, their ages ranged from 28 to 76 and they came from all walks of life.

I asked them to delve deeply and, in so doing, they uncovered old wounds but also excavated the healing tools that molded them into the women they are today. Interspersed among their spirited stories are essays with universal insights, light-hearted Notes to Self and guided journal questions for self-reflection.

My hope is that their courage may bolster you, their fears may dispel your own, their laughter may lighten you. Let their words be inscribed on your heart in indelible ink to illumine your own path. Welcome to the sisterhood whose markings we will always carry on our chests.

—Christy L. Schwan

Table of Contents

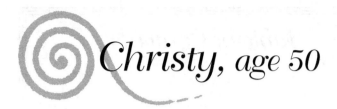# Christy, *age 50*

I 've been married over 30 years to the same thoughtful, gentle, considerate, impatient, exasperating man. We have two great children who both married individuals we would have chosen for them ourselves (if we'd been asked). We are indulgent grandparents to two-year old Madison Josephine, who stole our hearts the minute our daughter announced she was pregnant.

I would describe myself as strong, creative and challenge-oriented. My career has been centered in the insurance industry for the past 22 years and now I'm a partner in an all-female employee benefits consulting firm. My work is challenging and intense, requiring significant problem solving and persuasive skills. I love my work, our clients and the women who make up our organization.

My favorite color is yellow because it is vibrant, sunny, zesty, cheerful and warm. I'm a voracious reader and compulsive recipe collector, who loves to travel, explore new places, search for primitive antiques and take extended bike trips. I pamper myself with monthly pedicures and twice monthly massages. My life couldn't have been better on the day my cancer was diagnosed.

My first abnormal mammogram was around Halloween 2001—not what I was expecting in my trick or treat bag. I have no family history of breast cancer, so I was thrown off kilter immediately. To cope with the emotion and uncertainty, I kicked my take-charge, let's-get-this-over-and-done-with style into high gear. Two biopsies were completed quickly during the holiday season: the first, a stereotactic (needle) biopsy which confirmed my life-long dread of needles; the second, a lumpectomy with only a local anesthetic which eliminated my life-long fear of Valium.

A word to the uninitiated: Valium is your friend when undergoing local-anesthetic-only surgery. I didn't request, nor was I offered, Valium during either of my first two biopsies. The end result? I sobbed convulsively during both, couldn't stop shaking for about an hour after the surgeries were over, all the time apologizing to anyone who would listen that *"I am not a crier"*, *"I'm not an emotional person"*, *"I'm not a baby"* etc. I was surprised and embarrassed by my response and wish I'd asked for the Valium. I would have had less self-explaining to do.

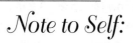

Note to Self:

Surgery isn't the time to be strong. Use any and all pharmaceutical crutches you need to help conserve your strength for recovery.

My first biopsy results came back with atypical cells only. My second biopsy was done the week between Christmas and New Year 2001. In the meantime, my family and friends were planning the celebration of my 50th birthday on New Year's Eve. One of the best presents I received that year was a gift certificate for a tattoo, something I'd always promised myself I'd get when I hit 50. (Yes, I know I hate needles, but a tattoo is different.) My son-in-law had researched tattoo artists and scheduled the appointment for early January before I could back out. I still didn't have the results back from the second biopsy when I had to make the decision about the design and placement of my tattoo.

The design decision was simple. I'm known as the "celestial being" in the office, so my choice of a moon and stars came easy. But placement was another issue. I'd always leaned toward my upper left breast, now the site of potential cancer. Then it hit me. Why waste a perfectly good tattoo if it turns out that I need to have a mastectomy? So my gorgeous blue and yellow moon and stars now sit safely on my back left shoulder blade. As it turned out, I had a year's reprieve before the cancer actually struck.

It's now March 2003 and I'm sitting here overlooking the Gulf of Mexico tapping away at my computer. I completed my radiation therapy a week ago and this is my reward—12 days in Clearwater, Florida (7 days alone with my husband followed by 5 days with our children, their spouses and our granddaughter). It's my celebration time for having made it across the abyss where the water and air are clearer than I've ever known, the colors are brighter, the laughter louder, the hugs tighter, the prayers calmer.

This is my breast cancer journey over the past year. My six-month post-biopsies mammogram showed no changes. By mid-November 2002, the calcifications in my left breast didn't look as good. A second stereoscopic biopsy revealed ductal carcinoma in situ (DCIS), the earliest form of detectable breast cancer, but cancer just the same. It was Friday morning, December 7th, when the nurse called me at my office to give me the news. At this point, I'd told no one other than my husband and my business partner, Lynn, about the latest series of tests. Anticipating further good news, I'd hoped to avoid telling anyone else at all. Although I immediately scheduled an appointment with the surgeon, I must have been in some weird form of denial, because it didn't hit me until my commute home that evening that I personally had cancer. That's when conscious vulnerability entered my life.

I'd always been strong, healthy, physically active with no medications and no significant injuries or illnesses other than knee surgery after sliding into first base during a softball game when I was 35. I had followed a healthy diet (all right, McDonald's french fries are my weekly weakness), I exercised regularly (all right, maybe just 3 days a week) and I rarely had more than one alcoholic drink per week (now that's the truth). How could cancer be growing in my body without my feeling anything? How could I have breast cancer when I breast fed my own babies? How could I have breast cancer when I had no family history of breast cancer? How could I have breast cancer when everything else in my life was going so well? How could, how could, how could…

I was presented with three choices by my medical advisors: a mastectomy, which they agreed was extreme considering the early stage at which my cancer was detected; a lumpectomy to remove the diseased area followed by radiation treatment; or watch and wait with quarterly mammograms. I chose the second path—lumpectomy with 7 weeks of radiation therapy. I know nearly two dozen women who've been faced with similar options and some chose the same path as I did, some made other choices, some even created their own unique list of options.

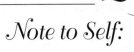

Note to Self:

Your treatment decision is one of the hardest multiple-choice questions you will ever answer, but the choice remains yours. There is more than one right answer, and the answer must fit your own personal path.

Dying was not my greatest fear—in fact, I wasn't afraid of dying at all. Perhaps because they found my cancer at such an early stage, I just couldn't imagine that I'd die from this encounter with breast cancer. I expect to live to be at least 95 and I didn't see this getting in my way.

My biggest fear was telling other people about my cancer because I wasn't sure I could handle their reactions. Initially, it was all I could do to keep myself together emotionally. I just couldn't deal with the concerns or emotional needs of others, not even my own children. My husband had to tell them and the other members of our family, although I did tell my parents and his. I also told my pastor and two of my closest friends who I knew could handle the news without unintentionally making me feel even more sad, or worse, sickly. I have an aversion to being viewed as frail, complaining or vulnerable. My business partner, who knew the details from Day 1, told everyone else, then assured me that if I were to lose my hair she would personally apply my false eyelashes and style my wig. Her reaction was exactly what I needed.

I realized how much easier it was to have the cancer myself rather than experience the anxiety and fear of having someone I love get cancer. Yet it was hard for me to let other people show concern, much less take care of me. I've always been the one others have turned to for help. I like being the rock, the one people count on for strength. I feared the pity I might see in other people's eyes if I let them come too close. Early on, a colleague stopped my one-woman march to self-sufficiency by quietly demanding, *"You have to let us in, you can't shut us out, you have to let us show you that we care about you even if you're uncomfortable with it."* So I gradually learned to get comfortable with it.

The low point for me was the day I went in to have the blue tattoos etched on my chest, to have a compressed foam body mold created, to get the coordinates calculated and to have a simulation run-through in preparation for the start of radiation. Since I'd been extremely healthy prior to this diagnosis, I certainly wasn't prepared for any of these procedures. All went fairly smoothly (what's another tattoo for a good cause?) until it came time for the CT scan machine, which I told myself looked like a big, harmless doughnut.

Now, I have issues with claustrophobia so I couldn't breathe once I was inside the doughnut. We tried an eye mask followed by relaxation techniques but I couldn't last five seconds, much less the five minutes the procedure required. The doctor advised a Valium but I'd planned to return to the office so I declined the offer. Plus, I was still wary of drugs at that point.

After several more futile attempts, I was near hysteria and crying uncontrollably so I agreed to half a Valium with the assurance that I'd still be able to drive myself back to the office for several more hours of work. That still didn't cut it. The medical technicians and doctor remained concerned and

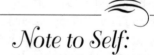

Note to Self:

Accept your limitations and know your areas of potential trauma. Try as many alternatives as you need and, if all else fails, set pride aside and go for the drugs.

compassionate, but they'd exhausted all of their options and recommended I reschedule that portion of my appointment. My self-preservation antenna signaled even higher anxiety with that alternative and instantly overrode my workaholic nature *"To hell with it, I'm not going back to the office. Give me the other half of the Valium."* And with that said, I relaxed enough to breathe through the procedure and allowed my husband to drive me home afterward.

I have to admit that experience heightened my sense of vulnerability and threw off the tenuous balance I'd created for myself. Although the actual radiation treatments lasted less than 3 minutes and were painless, I felt very fragile during that first week of treatment. Just walking into the treatment center made me so sad. The word *"cancer"* was everywhere: on the outside of the building, on the elevator, in the dressing room, on all of the brochures. For God's sake, it was even stamped on People magazine. In the waiting room, other patients there for treatment surrounded me. I never felt so alone in a room filled with so many people.

I couldn't get past my pervasive sadness, so I scheduled an appointment with the oncology psychologist. She helped me accept my tears, understand their source and develop a method for containing my emotion that would allow me to function fully on a day-to-day basis.

> ## *Note to Self:*
>
> *There is not a right way to experience cancer and its attendant emotions. If self-analysis fails you, seek professional advice and counsel. Even a couple of sessions can help you to realize you're normal.*

My feeling of vulnerability was stemming from the loss of control I had over my medical situation. To regain a sense of control, she suggested that I envision a box into which I would place all of my emotion for the week and then determine the time and frequency at which I would take it down off the shelf and allow it to be released. I immediately conjured up a deep purple cube about 12 inches across, with celestial symbols scrolled on all sides and decided that I would pull it down on Fridays, when another week of treatment was completed. That was all I needed to compartmentalize my emotion in a way that I could manage it. I didn't tell her that inside the box, entangled with all of my emotions, were Mardi Gras beads, feathered masks and gold doubloons.

My husband kept me going during the hard times. He lifted all household responsibilities off my shoulders so I could focus on my work and my recovery. He was able to sense when I needed to be left alone, when I needed a longer hug, when I needed to talk, when I needed to laugh and when I needed to cry. He didn't burden me with his emotion but allowed me the full range of my own. He took care of me without coddling, he never minimized my experience, he never once looked at me as though I was less than whole.

I grieved, though, each time I had to say, *"I have breast cancer."* I still grieve when I realize that my daughter and granddaughter will have to answer "Yes" when asked whether they have a family history of breast cancer.

Since I didn't need chemotherapy, I wasn't faced with side effects that kept me from continuing my full-time work schedule. That was important for my psyche and well-being in several ways: work kept my mind occupied; it kept me involved with other people; it made the time go faster; it held the sympathy from others at bay. Once radiation therapy started though, I did have to reduce my typical 10-hour workday down to 7 hours so I could make my daily 3:30 treatment. That was one appointment I was never late for, since I was concerned that if I missed a treatment I'd have to start all over again.

Note to Self:

No, you do NOT have to start over again if you miss an occasional treatment, but you do have to make it up, so it will push out the date of completion and your celebration party.

I went straight home after each treatment, put on my p.j.'s and became a couch slug (lower on the food chain than a potato). It was only at 4:30 p.m. each day that I would finally allow myself to submit to the reality of my situation and the growing fatigue about which I'd been forewarned. I've always loved a good nap, so I have to admit I began to look forward to my couch time. I'd get up long enough to eat the light supper my husband had fixed (he's petitioning for sainthood even though we're Lutheran) and then shuffle back to the couch.

Could I have continued to push myself through this period of treatment? Sure, but this was about and for me. I chose to take care of myself by being self-focused, self-protective and self-indulgent. At one point, my son succinctly and matter-of-factly acknowledged, *"Mom's on radiation and she doesn't have to do anything else she doesn't want to do."* For nearly two months, from 4:30 p.m. to 9:30 p.m. daily (at which time I got up and went to bed), I required nothing more of myself than the ability to assume a prone position nestled under a thick quilt in my very own family room. And it was good.

My daughter teased me that within 24 hours after my lumpectomy, I was on the phone placing a catalog shopping order. I remind her that it was just one week before Christmas and that she was the lucky recipient of many of the items ordered. She reminds me that I've never placed a catalog gift order without including something for myself. I remind her that I'm the mother and I can do whatever I want, especially when I was still facing radiation treatment. Conversation over.

On the other hand, someone commented (with good intentions I'm sure), *"Breast cancer is every woman's greatest nightmare. You must be having a terrible time accepting it."* I was stunned by her assumption. I'd personally never found my identity in my breasts prior to cancer and wasn't about to begin now. Since we aren't particularly close, I wrote it off as a comment made by someone who knew little about me.

My 7 weeks of daily radiation therapy began on a Thursday. I've always been a planner who likes setting and meeting milestones on a schedule, so I asked my assistant to purchase a roll of multi-colored metallic star-shaped stickers. After each therapy session, I affixed a star to both my calendar at work and at home. Actually, this was a re-creation of winning a star sticker for each spelling test that I got 100% on—one of my most vivid grade school memories.

When I began my star sticker ritual, I casually mentioned to my husband that this was a simple way for me to visually track my progress and to also celebrate the completion of another day of radiation. He wholeheartedly picked up on my need to celebrate milestones by sending a bouquet of flowers to my office every Wednesday (another week down, six to go…) throughout my treatment. Did I mention that the women in my office now refer to him as St. Paul? They would gather in my office for the weekly flower delivery and help me celebrate with their excitement. Other friends who knew about my treatment made it a point to either call me or think about me on Wednesdays. When I called one of them for a business reason early in the week, her first comment when she answered the phone was, *"It's not Wednesday, girl, so I'm not thinking about your boobs."*

Anointing my radiation-reddened skin with Aquaphor® became my morning and evening ritual, eliciting visceral memories of my mother's warm, healing touch when she smeared Vick's VapoRub® on our congested chests as kids—without the smell of menthol. I intentionally use the term anointing, because in time it began to feel like a spiritual ceremony: a ceremony whereby I was gentle with myself, where my own warm, soothing hands relieved some of the soreness, where I became familiar and comfortable with my own wounds and began to heal myself.

> ### *Note to Self:*
> *Insert your contact lenses prior to smoothing on the Aquaphor®, otherwise you'll end up having to remove, re-clean and reinsert your contacts several times throughout the day. The heavy ointment that works so well for healing plays havoc with contact lenses.*

At least once a week, I would reread the card my mother had sent me the day my cancer was diagnosed. Roy Lessin penned these words:

Always Remember

Always remember,
when God made you
He did so with a purpose and a plan.
He saw all your days before you lived one of them
and placed over you the covering of his protective love.
He has allowed nothing to come into your life that has
not first been screened through that love.
His hand has remained upon you to this very day.
He calls you by name.
You are his beloved child…
the apple of His eye…
the delight of His heart.
Today you are in the exact place He wants you to be,
and tomorrow He will be with you as He has always been—
in goodness, in kindness, in faithfulness.

But it's these simple words written by my mother that gave me the quiet assurance and strength I needed: *You are in our thoughts and prayers constantly! You are strong and healthy. I know you are going to be OK. Love, Mother*

After my last day of radiation, my husband steered me into the living room and began a rambling, disjointed explanation of the theme he'd chosen for the celebration. Somehow it involved freedom: freedom from therapy, freedom to live my life without the fear of cancer, freedom to live a long life. He was shaking with excitement when he presented me with my very own… Harley Davidson 100th anniversary leather jacket! You need to understand that my husband is not just an HD aficionado—he's a true zealot. This was the best possible gift he could ever imagine giving me. I have to agree it was a great way to commemorate the year my treatment ended since it coincided with Harley's 2003 birthday. Oh yeah, he'd also hidden a diamond solitaire necklace in one of the zippered pockets. (The Pope's U.S. emissaries have been calling.)

Our children joined us for a celebratory dinner that evening. My business partner hand-mosaiced, in all my favorite colors, a seven-step spiral ladder to honor the occasion. My best friend sent a firecracker-hued bouquet of flowers in red, orange, purple and yellow. And I added the final gold star to my calendar.

So what have I learned from all of this? I learned that illness does not equal frailty, that courage does not come without tears, that compassion is not the same as pity, that the laughter lasts longer than the pain, that letting people in lets the emotion out.

I learned that once people know you have breast cancer, they reveal their own bout with the disease. I learned that nearly everyone knows at least half a dozen other women who have encountered breast cancer. I learned that many women are anxious to tell their own story—sometimes as a warning, sometimes as a catalyst, always as a catharsis.

The most unexpected gift I received was learning how many people cared about me. Whether they called, sent a note, stopped me in the hall, added me to their prayer list, squeezed my arm or just kept me in their thoughts, I've never been told I was loved more frequently than during this period of my life nor have I expressed it more often myself. There's something about a sudden, critical health condition that brings out the need to say *"I love you."*

Someone once said that a life-threatening illness can be a mentor in your life if you allow it. Breast cancer changed the balance in my life, giving more importance to some things and less to others. Breast cancer taught me to be gentle with myself, it showed me how to let other people in and thereby deepened my relationships. It also led me back to my writing.

Breast cancer changed the balance in my life, giving more importance to some things and less to others.

In an odd way, breast cancer relaxed me. My innate need to control situations was stopped dead in its tracks. How could I control something that I didn't even know I had? Once I did know, I could make decisions, but I still couldn't control the outcome. Giving up? No way! But accepting my inability to control outcomes was a revelation that permeates my entire life. *"Lord, help me"* and *"Lord, protect me"* became my serenity prayers. Those silent three-word petitions were all I needed to feel God's calming presence no matter where I was at the time.

I will always remember Tia, the valet parking attendant at Columbia Hospital's Cancer Care Center. Our lives couldn't have been more different, yet she expressed her concern daily with a simple, genuine, non-intrusive, *"How ya doing today, Christy?"* and thereby helped me to re-center myself. Our short exchanges lengthened as the days went by and she was as joyful as I on my last day of treatment. Even though I was just one of dozens of patients she saw each day, I felt her personal touch and was calmed by her gentle compassion. She was as much a healing presence to me as the radiation therapists and my oncology doctor.

With my mother, my sister, my daughter and granddaughter, I hope to walk in the Race for the Cure for years to come. And I will celebrate every March 10th as a day of completion, commemoration, and freedom. My plans are simple… gathering my family around me while adding another gold star to my calendar.

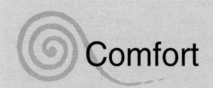 # Comfort

Some women find comfort in journaling about their experiences and feelings as they go through treatment. Some women receive value meeting with other women in a structured support group environment. Some women turn to a close circle of family and/or friends for all they want and need. Some women prefer to go it alone, relying on their own internal resources.

The first and last entry in my breast cancer journal stated: *"Ok, so it's the first day of my radiation treatment. 1 down, 34 to go. Pretty manageable, only one needle, no claustrophobic episodes, no pain. So, that's all I want to say about it. I'm in the countdown."*

I couldn't, wouldn't, didn't write more than that until my treatment was completed. Creativity, introspection, insight fell off my radar—my writing ability seemed to evaporate.

I went to only one breast cancer support group meeting. The mixture of fearfulness and vulnerability mingled with forced optimism and cheerfulness was too much for me. I couldn't, wouldn't, didn't want to meet new people in the context of my breast cancer.

But like a starved prisoner, I began to write voraciously once my treatment was completed. I'd missed the self-reflection, self-realization, self-release, maybe even self-redemption that writing gave me. From there, I began to reach out to women who had been touched by breast cancer. I talked with women from the support group meeting, from church, from work, from the neighborhood. And then they introduced me to their friends and families. Their words became a comforting quilt that wrapped warmly around me. I wish the same warmth for you as you read their stories.

—*Christy L. Schwan*

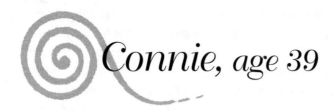

Connie, *age 39*

*C*onnie has been married to her high school sweetheart, Todd, for almost 18 years. Self- described as caring, somewhat controlling, and nurturing, she and her husband co-own an insurance agency with his parents. Connie works part-time as the bookkeeper and also keeps very busy running her two teen-age daughters back and forth to school and other events. Basically, they were a very faith-filled, contented, happy family until June 2002.

On Tuesday, June 11, Connie went to her family doctor for her annual physical. She felt better than she had in ten years since she'd lost quite a bit of weight the year before and was feeling very healthy. He proceeded with her exam and right away felt something in her left breast at the 2 o'clock position. The look in his eyes told her something was wrong. Everything seemed fine in her right breast, but he gave her a referral for a mammogram to check out the small lump he'd found on the left side. Although he was not overly concerned, Connie was already nervous. *"I went in feeling great and came out feeling like I'd been hit by a semi."*

Once home, she immediately called to schedule the mammogram and was told it would be two weeks before they could see her. She lost it. No way was she going to wait two weeks. She had a hard lump in her breast! She called a second time and explained the situation to another woman but was again told that the wait would be two weeks. The next morning without her knowledge, Todd called and "convinced" them to squeeze her in two days later. Connie doesn't know what he said, did or promised, but their persistence paid off.

The radiologist was rightfully alarmed when she read the mammogram, so she immediately took an ultrasound. Fairly certain that it was a cancerous tumor, she then performed a needle punch biopsy, the results of which would not come until the following week. Connie's family doctor called her on the following Monday afternoon to tell her that the biopsy was positive for cancer. *"I felt like I couldn't breathe. I had a sick feeling all weekend but until I knew for sure, I was hoping and praying for it to be negative. I had no family history, nursed both my babies, did not drink or smoke and was not overweight, although I did eat an occasional Big Mac."*

The next few days were a whirlwind of appointments with her family doctor, the surgeon, and the oncologist. Because the tumor was very fast growing, they concurred that a lumpectomy followed by chemotherapy followed by radiation would be the best course of treatment. They were guessing that it was Stage 1 but couldn't be sure until after the surgery. Connie's

Note to Self:

After you hear the word "cancer", you don't hear much after that for a while. It helps to have a second or third set of ears to hear when yours aren't functioning well.

sister-in-law was visiting from out-of-state during this time and went with Connie and Todd to every doctor visit in the beginning.

Then they hit another stumbling block—the surgeon was booked solid for six weeks. Connie couldn't imagine leaving the aggressive tumor growing inside of her for that long, but the only way they could fit her in was if someone else cancelled their surgery. Connie called her cousin, who called his father (a noted heart doctor), who called her surgeon, who called Connie to say she would be first on the waiting list if a cancellation occurred. Connie prayed so fervently for an open door (realizing that she was trying to take another woman's slot) that one day she ran right through a stoplight. *"The first of many prayers were answered at 4:30 that afternoon, when they called to say I could have my surgery on July 1st. Another woman had decided to delay her breast reconstruction."*

As a former medical assistant, Connie's natural instinct was *"Show me the lab reports and the mammogram films, explain the terms, give me all the details."* She would never just take the doctor's word for it.

Even with answered prayers, Connie just couldn't stop crying during the three weeks prior to her surgery. Faced with the cancer diagnosis, Connie automatically thought of death but was never afraid of it. Her personal faith kept her going. Plus at 39 she was certain that she wasn't ready to leave yet. But she was afraid of the unknown, being the type of person who likes answers, likes to take care of things immediately and wants to know things NOW!

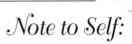

Note to Self:

Pushy, persuasive, demanding, insistent, convincing, relentless, persistent—whatever adjective it takes, use it. A diagnosis of cancer is not the time to be demure. Ask for favors. Ask for exceptions. Ask all the questions you need to. Ask for forgiveness later.

As a wife and mother, she worried most about her family—her husband and her daughters. *"Who's going to make sure they have their lunch money everyday? Who's going to pick them up after school and run them to their activities? Who's going to wash their sheets and clothes? Who's going to…"* The sadness and uncertainty were nearly crushing her.

She reached her lowest point a few days before the surgery. She was filled with worry and felt like she was losing control. *"I remember going to my bedroom one evening sobbing. I knelt in prayer and told God that I needed him now more than ever. 'Please be with me and take away my fears', I prayed. The next day was different, I wasn't consumed with worry. The night before my surgery, I felt peace for the first time in many weeks. God gave me the rest I needed."*

The first words out of Connie's mouth after surgery were, *"What about my lymph nodes?"* With a big smile, her husband told her that the sentinel node biopsy showed that all three of the removed nodes were cancer-free. Gratefully relieved, Connie learned that the entire waiting room was filled with church members gathered for a prayer vigil.

Although the tumor was fairly small, the oncologist was concerned that it was estrogen negative and very aggressive. She described it as a *"nasty"* tumor that would require a harsh chemotherapy regimen— four treatments each three weeks apart. Connie had a bad reaction to the anti-nausea drug after her first treatment. It made her so jittery and agitated that she couldn't eat, read or sleep. Feeling like she was tied up in knots with no way to escape, she finally called her doctor. Once he switched her medication she felt much better. She just wished she'd called sooner.

Connie's scalp became tender and sore almost as soon as the chemo began; her hair began to fall out eleven days later. It was the next hardest thing to hearing the initial diagnosis of cancer. Being the get-it-done-right-now person she is, Connie called her good friend and hairdresser, who came over first thing the next morning and buzzed

> ### *Note to Self:*
> *Tears will come, sooner or later. Let them flow, let them wash over you, let them find their own healing course. No dam(n) can hold them back permanently.*

off all her hair. *"Everyone said I looked like Demi Moore in GI Jane. That was until all my hair, even the stubble, fell out. Then I looked like Mr. Clean. I lost every eyelash and eyebrow. I felt crappy and looked like a pale, shiny alien. I cried and cried and cried."* For Connie, each look in the mirror was an inescapable reminder of her cancer.

She'd gone to the wig store with her mother, daughters and a friend prior to her hair loss, when the trip could be more relaxed and less rushed. Although everyone tried to be cheerful, it was an undeniably depressing day. *"I can't believe this is happening to me,"* filled her heart and mind.

Connie did feel fortunate that she lost her hair when the weather was cooler; otherwise, her wig would have been itchy and hot. She wore her wig whenever she went out, wanting to look "normal", not wanting people to look at her and think, *"Oh, look. She's got cancer."* She did buy several hats and bandannas though, her favorite being a soft, comfortable, pink terry cloth cap. With a smile, she admits that she never had a bad-hair day with her wig and it was certainly less time-consuming, since it never had to be blown dry or styled.

Connie was bald during Halloween, so when she and a good friend were discussing potential costumes, it was only natural that her friend blurted out, *"You'd make a great Casper the Ghost!"*

Each round of chemo made Connie progressively weaker, so she chose not to go to work during the duration of her treatments. She lay on the couch for 3 to 4 days after each chemo; her worst days were the Fridays after the Wednesday treatments. Her mother stayed with her and cared for her during those tough times. Her mother-in-law, friends and neighbors brought in dinner on those days.

Even with all that great country cooking and the steroids in the chemo making her hungry, she had no appetite. Nothing sounded good except for the homemade potato soup that one of her neighbors brought over one day. *"I still think about that soup and the little lemon cake with a powdered-sugar-etched heart on the top. Those were the best gifts ever."*

> ### *Note to Self:*
> *It's surprising who calls and who doesn't. People handle crises differently. If they don't call or reach out, it doesn't mean they don't care. They just may not know how to show it.*

Her third round of chemo was the worst, with indescribable fatigue and irritability for 4 to 5 days after. The doctor had to do some heavy talking to convince Connie to continue with the fourth and final treatment. With positive self-talk and prayerful petitions, Connie finished her chemo and moved on to radiation. *"Three weeks after chemo, I was happy to start radiation—33 treatments, five days a week for 6 1/2 weeks. Radiation was a walk in the park compared to chemo."*

Connie didn't attend any formal cancer support group meetings, but she did get to know the other women as they waited in line for their radiation. While sad to be among that group of women, it was also heartening to see how each was coping with her own situation. It wasn't unusual for someone to readily open up her gown, exclaim with unselfconscious abandon, *"Look at me!"* to show the others specifically how she was doing. Others would lift up their wigs and compare hair growth—hope growing along with their hair. It was a sorority like none other.

Driving to and from treatments was Connie's quiet time for reflection and prayer. It became a daily ritual to pray for herself and the other women she'd met.

Even though he, too, was scared, Todd's upbeat attitude, strength and faith kept Connie going. Todd would hold her, cry with her, talk when she needed to talk, listen to her complain about her bald head and tell her she was still beautiful. *"But the most memorable times, the times I hold closest in my heart, are the walks we took along our quiet country road. We'd stop, hold each other and pray out loud together in the middle of that road with the cornfields on either side. There's just something about that road that still fills me with a calming, centering peace.*

"My last treatment was on my 40th birthday, December 2, 2002. What a celebration! It was the end of a sad six months and I felt like a bird let out of its cage. My entire family met us for dinner and birthday cake. I was actually happy to be turning 40. The best part is, I never have to be 39 again!"

Connie's next step was throwing out the creams and ointments she'd used during her treatments. *"That*

Note to Self:

Some dates will never be forgotten: the date the lump was found, the date of diagnosis, the date of surgery, the date chemo began and ended, the date radiation began and ended. They are recorded forever on your mind, body and spirit.

hospital smell was a reminder I didn't need. But I did keep every card and I received hundreds, some days 10 to 20, many from people I hardly knew." And to complete the circle, on the first anniversary of her surgery, Todd sent a thank-you card to the surgeon.

"I would say my life gifts were the prayers of so many people. People I didn't even know said they were praying for me. I was on several prayer chains on the Internet. It was truly overwhelming. My eyes still tear up thinking about the well wishes I received.

"I learned that in the past, I tried to rely on others or myself for guidance instead of relying on the Lord. This experience has taught me to be more patient and to leave painful times in God's hands. It has taught me to think about myself less and others more. I feel I am much more compassionate to other's needs. I'm saddened to hear of anyone experiencing cancer, chemo, pain and loss."

Connie grieves every time she tells someone about her breast cancer and every time she meets another woman with the disease. She grieves for her daughters who will have this worry upon them because of a family history. *"My priorities have changed. I used to LOVE to shop. New clothes and shoes just don't bring as much excitement as they used to. And you know what? Boobs aren't important to me anymore either."* Todd walks by at this point in our conversation and inserts, *"I agree… partially."*

"I'm looking for more meaning in my life and I'm considering volunteer work with other cancer patients." Without realizing it, Connie has already developed a ritual of Passing the Hats. She has shared her rainbow collection of hats with two other family friends who've since developed breast cancer.

"I live one day at a time and count my blessings, even the small ones. I know I had breast cancer for a reason. Maybe it was to make me more compassionate. I am. Maybe it was to let my Lord have more control in my life. I have. Maybe it was to make me talk to Him more. I do.

"I totally and completely cherish my husband and daughters. Todd has been the love of my life for so long (since we were fifteen) that I can't imagine my life without him. Every minute of every hour I have with him is even more special because I truly realize that it could have been taken away. I want to see my girls grow up and marry the man of their dreams just as I did."

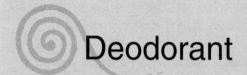Deodorant

Yesterday I cleaned out the drawers of my bathroom vanity. I'd purchased several bright white plastic drawer organizers and was determined that I would finally toss all of my outdated cosmetic samples, wrong-hued-never-worn lipsticks, old contact lens cases, and hair products that had turned my natural curls into a literal frizz-bomb. As I cold-heartedly filled the wastebasket, I came upon the organic, all natural, lavender-scented deodorant. Twice I tossed it and twice I retrieved it.

I think back to the day I'd made the purchase, stopping by Outpost Foods on my way home from the hospital. I can't remember the exact day or whether I'd already started radiation therapy or not. I just remember combing the aisles of the unfamiliar store, not wanting to ask for help, finally finding several alternatives without the forbidden aluminum chlorohydrate (which can interfere with radiation) and being unable to make up my mind. Standing there alone, I was suddenly overwhelmed with the choices confronting me. Or is affronting the better word? Unable to decide, I bought sample sizes of them all and figured that should last me through the seven weeks of radiation treatments.

I recall each morning putting Secret Platinum Protection Powder Fresh Anti-Perspirant under my right arm and then religiously applying the organic, all natural, lavender-scented deodorant under my left. I'd settled fairly quickly on that option for two reasons: purple is my favorite color and I thought the scent did the best job of minimizing underarm odor, at least temporarily. Fleeting thoughts spilled out of me with each application. *"I don't care what the package proclaims. I know this won't do the job. Why does this stupid cancer have to impact my personal hygiene options? Who's gonna know if I use my Secret today? What am I complaining about, at least I don't need chemo."* And finally, with resignation, *"I know this, too, will pass."*

The morning after the completion of radiation therapy, I smeared an extra thick, luxuriant layer of Secret under my left armpit. Breathing deeply, I could feel the powder freshness down to my toes and briefly considered sending a testimonial letter to Proctor & Gamble. It's been six months now since that day. My six-month mammogram came back looking fine, although it was the most painful one I've ever had. The nurse later told me that healing takes several months, so the pain wasn't unusual, just unexpected on my part.

Unexpected. Unsuspecting. What innocence, what naïveté is buried in those words. My husband and I just returned from our end-of-summer vacation "up north". Driving back, I realized that a year ago at this time I had no inkling that cancerous cells were growing within my body. No hint, no clue, no premonition, no hunch, no sign. I thought about what I didn't know last year, what I've been through, and what I know now. I thought about what I don't know now that I will know next year. And then I stopped thinking because I was moving into scary territory.

I carefully replaced the organic, all natural, lavender-scented deodorant in a corner of the bright white plastic drawer organizer in my bathroom vanity. Its lavender-colored cap a visual reminder of my radiation treatment, as are the scars on my left breast. Through the clutter of daily living, I'm sure the deodorant will eventually be shoved towards the back of the drawer, where it will again lay unnoticed and unused. But at some point, perhaps the next time I reorganize, I will unexpectedly pull it out again and take the time to reflect on what I do and don't know then.

—Christy L. Schwan

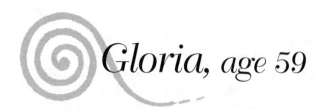

Gloria, age 59

Quiet and reserved, Gloria warms up best in one-to-one conversations. Home, family and tradition are the most important things in her life (other than golf, which she started playing in her 50s.) She fulfilled a long-held dream by gifting herself with piano lessons after retirement. Her two sons often tease her about her naïveté. In turn, she cuts out articles to prove she knows what she's talking about.

She was just thirteen when her mother died of uterine cancer. So her sister, Janette, who is ten years older, became her surrogate mother. Growing up, they shared everything, including a bedroom. Now 68 and retired from her marketing position for a major newspaper, Gloria reflects back on her cancer experience.

"It was just a routine mammogram with the usual pinching, compressing and momentary uncomfortable feeling, or so I thought. I was not prepared for the phone call from the radiologist asking me to come in for a few more pictures and a possible ultrasound. Oh dear! The heart is starting to race a little and the fear factor is creeping in. Didn't my sister, Janette, receive the very same call six years ago? Aren't we like twins, despite our age difference? We share many of the same attributes and genes. We're both soft-spoken and family-oriented. We travel and vacation well together, and even wear the same color and style clothing to family gatherings. We share our illnesses, too. What she has had I know I will get seven to ten years down the line. Are we to share this, too?"

Additional tests, the long wait and then the phone call from the radiologist. *"We suggest you contact a surgeon to discuss a possible biopsy."* Appointment made, films reviewed, choices given: wait and see (after all, most of these lumps turn out to be benign) or perform a biopsy on her right breast. Sensing that the surgeon opted for the latter, Gloria agreed. *"The surgery turned out to be a lumpectomy. I was conscious during the procedure, but in La La land and remember the surgeon saying, 'Boy, am I glad we did this.' I knew this meant cancer."* Additional tissue was removed, sent to the lab for testing and then more waiting.

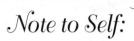

> ## *Note to Self:*
> *Hearing becomes acute while in La La land. Side comments can last in our memories forever.*

The call came to confirm what Gloria already sensed—it was indeed cancer. *"I was home from work that day and alone. I was numb, scared and overwhelmed. Ahead lay appointments and discussions with the surgeon, oncologist and radiation oncologist. Emotions were on a roller coaster ride. LOWS: How should I plan for the time I have left? Will I see my grandchildren grow up? Was it the estrogen in those birth control pills I took for so many years? How will my husband ever find his socks and underwear without me? Oh, such morbid thoughts. HIGHS: Didn't Janette recover from her breast cancer? Mine was just a small lump, wasn't it? I didn't need chemotherapy, did I? There must be others who have been through this. The beautiful and popular TV weather girl has it too; even the rich and famous can't escape this disease."*

Her surgeon was very supportive, taking Gloria under her wing and helping her throughout the process. The cancer was caught early and the lump was small, but it was still hard for Gloria to admit that something was wrong with her. *"I'd never even had a cold before this. I was close-mouthed about my fears and instead tried to find the reason for it: what triggered it, where did it come from, what I'd done wrong. My husband had a difficult time handling it and didn't talk about it. I comforted him. He did express his fears to our sons; they were positive and comforting for both of us.*

"I read books and magazine articles and felt very sorry for myself initially. It seemed the more I discovered, the more depressed I became. Invasive cancer, DCIS, Flow Cytometry, estrogen receptors, metastasis—what does all this mean? Support groups weren't for me—too many people with too many fears. I decided to let God take care of things and be as optimistic as possible. The women are the rocks in our family. I turned to my sister who gave me all I needed. She passed her good attitude on to me and helped me see that this was just another phase of life I had to go through."

The hardest step for Gloria was telling her close-knit group of co-workers. Their compassion bolstered her as she cried for the first time about her diagnosis.

The radiation routine began: up at 5 a.m. for a 7 a.m. radiation treatment, then to work by 8 a.m. It was a routine that kept her busy and let her maintain a level of normalcy. Her husband, who was already retired at the time, faithfully drove her to and from appointments and work each day. After seven weeks, it was over with only a little skin redness and a sore rotator cuff due to the awkward arm position required. No special celebrations. Just relief and a readiness to move on now that the treatments were behind her.

> *Note to Self:*
> Relief is a celebration.
> Moving on is a celebration.
> Party hats aren't necessary.

"Tamoxifen became the pill of the day: two each day for five years. Janette doesn't do this. Should I worry? No. Keep positive. Keep active. Keep praying. The word cancer slips into the back of my mind only to resurface at each six-month mammogram. Finally, the magic number—five years! I'm safe! But my sister wasn't so lucky. Six months after my diagnosis, Janette found a lump, this time on the right side. Her cancer was more complicated than mine and required chemotherapy as well as radiation. Now it was my turn to listen, comfort and support. We are in it together."

Gloria had just passed her sixth year of being cancer free when the call came again after her annual mammogram—more pictures and a possible biopsy. *"Here we go again. Left side. I should have known—just following in my sister's footsteps. Guess that Tamoxifen didn't do the trick for me. Well, I sure know the routine anyway. The surgeon is recommending the usual lumpectomy along with a new procedure looking for a sentinel lymph node using a dye injected into the body. OK, if that's what's happening now, even though I sometimes feel like a guinea pig.*

"After hours of searching, mine couldn't be found. Maybe I didn't have one of those? Rather than take out the usual dozen or more nodes, I asked the surgeon to look around for that sentinel and if it couldn't be found in the first three or four, forget it. My sister had some problems with Lymphedema and I didn't want any part of that. The four or five nodes the surgeon removed were cancer free, so I'm hopeful this was the right decision."

More radiation, but this time Gloria was able to have treatments at a hospital closer to home. She'd recently retired and was able to drive herself to appointments. In typical male fashion, her husband plotted out the best route to get there with the least traffic and fewest stop lights. *"I was one of the first patients in their new radiology center. I just prayed that they weren't practicing on me! The radiation technicians were great at making me feel comfortable and complimented my surgeon's handiwork, 'Oh, she did a really good job on you!' but I would have preferred a rose tattoo or something a little more decorative this time. I followed my husband's route on the way there, but since I didn't have to hurry to get to work after my treatments, I'd meander on my way home, stopping by a few rummage sales."*

> ### ᐰote to Self:
> *Meandering as a form of healing? Maybe the best trips are those that aren't the shortest or fastest route between two places.*

Gloria compares her cancer recurrence to golfing. *"If my first hole is horrible, I always tell myself that the next hole has to be better. You can't have two bad holes in a row, so doing poorly on the first hole can be a good thing. You can still end up having a great game."*

She continues to check for early warning signals, but she's also more aware of the life and people around her. She's more likely to reach out to others because she appreciated what others did for her during her treatments. *"My husband belongs to the Shriners and the wives usually only get together quarterly. Prior to my cancer diagnosis, we didn't have much to say to each other. There were at least ten to fifteen breast cancer survivors who circled around me once they found out. It's like a buried treasure of other women, an informal support group, a special club. We greet each other with a heartfelt, 'How are you doing?' Not a casually polite 'How are you?' We genuinely want to know how each other is coming along."*

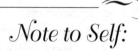

Note to Self:

Buried treasure is uncovered just by reaching out to other survivors. No digging required.

Gloria now has about eight months left of her five-year regimen of Arimidex, a drug that has fewer side effects than Tamoxifen. *"I'm down to yearly mammograms again. The first two years were a little unsettling. Each time the six-month mammogram was done, I required additional pictures of suspicious areas and a biopsy. I wonder if a cancer patient is ever free of the specter that hides in the back of our minds. Will it come again, next time in a different area—the bones, liver, brain? Just two years ago, my sister-in-law, cancer free for twenty years, discovered a lump in her remaining breast. The lump proved to be cancerous and required a second mastectomy. I cannot worry about my tomorrow. I must refrain from checking the death notices, looking for cancer as the cause of death and noting the age of the women. Having breast cancer is no longer the death threat of decades ago. Hope is on the horizon. I use my spiritual faith for personal growth and look for the blessings life is holding for me."*

What Cancer Cannot Do

Cancer is so limited...
It cannot cripple Love
It cannot shatter Hope
It cannot corrode Faith
It cannot destroy Peace
It cannot kill Friendship
It cannot suppress Memories
It cannot silence Courage
It cannot invade the Soul
It cannot steal eternal Life
It cannot conquer the Spirit
—Author Unknown

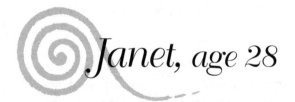

Janet, age 28

I first met Janet at a breakfast meeting to rally volunteers for an upcoming breast cancer benefit walk. As one of the keynote speakers, Janet spoke briefly but candidly about her breast cancer experience at the age of 28. I knew I needed to include her story as she talked about playing the cancer card when she needed an extra measure of consideration or as an easy way to get out of doing something she didn't want to do.

Now 32, Janet is a single, outgoing, youngest-of-four-kids, purposeful, statuesque blonde who became the family and friend social planner at an early age. She's not above "fake snakes on camping trips" goofiness. She's very close to her family and has built a raft of long-term relationships. As a recreational therapist working in a senior facility, Janet helps patients regain their vitality by bringing back fun activities into their lives. What led her to this field? She says it was her interest in health care coupled with the closeness she'd always felt for her grandfather.

Her doctor found the lump in her left breast during her annual physical. Janet's unease was immediate. There was no family history of breast cancer, but a 29-year-old friend had just been diagnosed. The subsequent mammogram came back clear, but the doctor was still concerned. So he ordered an ultrasound which revealed the lump. A stereotactic biopsy was performed in late November as Christmas music played in the background. Friends drove her to her parent's house afterward.

"On December 1st, the surgeon called to tell me that it was Stage 2 cancer. His first words were, 'We didn't know who should tell you.' My other doctors were either on vacation or unavailable, yet they didn't want me to hear the news from someone I didn't know. He was the designated caller.

"At twenty-eight, I was terrified that if I didn't take aggressive action it would come back. I wanted to get rid of it, get it over with and move on with my life. I asked many of my friends, both male and female, what they would do. Within three days, my family and I met with the surgeon, the oncologist and the plastic surgeon. I decided to have a bi-lateral mastectomy and the surgery was scheduled for December 12th. My mom ended up telling everyone in her annual Christmas card. I'd been planning a Christmas party for work, so a lot of people were freaked out by the news. It's weird when someone with my energy level is diagnosed.

"The surgeon and oncologist explained everything to me, but my appointment with the plastic surgeon was anguishing. One of his first comments was, 'Aren't you excited?' His practice had obviously been primarily with patients electing cosmetic surgery, not reconstructive

surgery. I was sobbing the entire time and he didn't know how to handle it.

"I became so mad, so angry. It was so unfair. I didn't do anything to deserve this. I didn't want to scare anyone, but I didn't know what to do with my anger. I screamed at my doctors, 'You're going to make me this bitter woman.' Inside, I was agonizing. Will I ever be fun again? As a single woman, I wondered if anyone would ever be able to understand."

Determined to maintain her social life, Janet and a friend went to hear a local bar band play the week after her diagnosis. After a fun night, they were halfway home when her friend mistakenly turned the wrong way down a one-way street. When the police sirens wailed, Janet's first response was, *"This is all I need,"* as she instinctively reached for the cancer card. She didn't have to use it (the officers just gave them a warning), but the cancer card had been activated and was ready for service.

The day of surgery her whole family was in the room. Everyone else was nervous. Janet remained calm, *"I knew I couldn't move on with my life until I'd taken care of the cancer."* The oncologist initially thought it was DCIS and a single lump. During surgery, a second lump was discovered along the chest wall, confirming that she'd made the right decision regarding mastectomy. The first step in reconstruction was also taken; expanders were inserted to help her skin stretch for the future implants.

When she arrived at her parents' home after surgery, they'd covered all of their mirrors with newspapers so that she could only see her face. But Janet was OK with her scars and the paper quickly came down. Janet stayed with her parents for a month. *"That was a real comfort. Our daily ritual was to sit side-by-side on the couch and open all of the cards I'd received. I'd read a card and cry, pass it to Mom and then she'd read it and cry. A loving but typical male, my dad was bewildered and kept asking, 'We're OK! Why are we crying?'"*

As a special treat, one of her college friends offered to come and help Janet wash her hair. It made Janet feel like a little kid, yet she couldn't do it herself since she still had a limited range of arm motion. A mutually beneficial act of compassion, it was wonderful to be pampered and have her hair washed, blown dry and styled. Her friend felt great about it, since it was the one unique favor she could do for Janet.

"I didn't struggle with chemo so I continued to work full-time. A port was put in on the first day and I only felt sick after the first treatment. But I did have a hard time whenever I entered the cancer ward. I'd stare straight ahead and never look at anyone. These people were so sick and I just couldn't accept that I was one of them. For every chemo session, my brother came and sat with me over his lunch hour. Then I'd spend the days after each chemo treatment at my parent's house—they were my backbone of strength. My mom became my personal secretary and went with me to all of my appointments. We've always been close and she still wants to be right there for all of my follow-up appointments. She's become super-protective and can now be hypercritical of anyone I'm dating. She wants the perfect person for me."

With the four Taxol treatments, Janet did have joint pain, which at times was so severe she'd have to leave in the middle of a staff meeting. Her doctor had given her a prescription for Percocet to relieve the pain but she'd stoically refused it until he finally confronted her with, *"Quit being a martyr and just take it!"*

During physical therapy exercise, Janet's favorite song was *"Who I Am"* by Jessica Andrews. It was a reminder that she was still the same Janet, even though her body was going through so much. *"My physical therapist was the best part of treatment and she quickly became my counselor as well. My mom and I thought I'd been doing fine with my exercises, but my therapist's first reaction was 'You need a lot of help.' It was exciting to see my daily progress and how quickly I improved with her guidance. When I could finally raise my arm above my head again, we were both thrilled. I realized then how easy it is to take the little things for granted.*

"There are certain parts of myself I treasure; my long, blond hair was one of them. Before my hair fell out, I had a Shaving Party. I figured that these were the people who were going to see me bald anyway, so of course they weren't going to say I looked bad. I was right—everyone thought I looked great, especially my mom. She kept saying 'Your head is so round!' Then she told my friends and me that when I was born, mothers were advised to keep changing their baby's sleeping positions, so that their heads wouldn't get flat on one side. We still laugh that my mom was so proud she had done such a good job! Most mothers never get to see the results of their frequent baby-turning. Once my hair was gone, I was OK with it. Afterwards, people would ask me if I was wearing a wig or whether it was my real hair. I was OK with that, too."

Halfway through chemo, a friend planned a Bead & Blessing Party. All of the women that Janet loved came over, each bringing a unique bead. As they encircled her, they each offered a bead along with a blessing or story about how she had touched their lives. It was a tear-filled, yet joyful evening and boosted her spirit for the remaining treatments. Janet received enough beads to make both a necklace and a watch that she still loves to wear.

Note to Self:

It is a close women's circle that surrounds you once you're diagnosed with breast cancer.

Included in that group was her mother's best friend from high school, who was undergoing treatment for breast cancer at the same time. She offered precious support to both Janet and her mother and attended the party even though it was held on her own birthday. She died just a few months later.

There were some people who backed away during her treatment. Janet admits that it felt like a personal attack. *"I'm an avid baseball and volleyball player and continued to play even when I was bald. The first couple of games I wore I wig and a hat. The pitcher, who I had considered a friend, just couldn't deal with it. My reaction? I started wearing a scarf only. My way of saying, 'So there!' I realized it had been a surface friendship only.*

"Emotionally, I felt like I'd fallen down a hole. While everyone else was getting married and having babies, I was dealing with cancer. I grieved for what I thought I missed out on. I attended a couple of support group meetings but struggled because my issues were so different; dating and fertility were my concerns.

"Eventually, I attended a Mind, Body, Spirit workshop at Stillwaters Center. The leader taught me how to get my thoughts on paper so she could help me, even though I'm not a journal-keeper. I made a list of all the reasons I should live and the beautiful things people said about me. I was particularly worried about how and when to tell a guy, so I wrote a letter to a 'future boyfriend' that was very healing. I also wrote a letter to a friend who had pulled away and let me down, although I never gave it to her."

During treatment she was dating someone who had a Harley and finally had to tell him why she couldn't ride—fear of losing her wig in the wind. The relationship didn't last but Janet doesn't think it was just the cancer. *"I haven't had to worry about it as much as I thought. I gave a copy of the letter to my current boyfriend after we'd dated about two months so he could understand why I'd made my choices. It was a very tender moment for both of us."*

That summer, her brother was married. He and his fiancé had just started planning their wedding when Janet was diagnosed. Janet was a proud bridesmaid. Bald at the time, she wore her wig and had her former eyebrows penciled in. *"As I was walking down the aisle, I kept thinking how happy I was to be here. I was thankful that I looked and felt normal and wasn't the center of attention. It was their day and I didn't want to take it away from them. Since then, I've shown wedding pictures to some of my boyfriends who've commented on how hot I looked—fake hair, fake eyebrows and all!"*

Janet's email name is "extremejanet". An apt description for sure! Janet has always celebrated her young nephews' birthdays by taking them for a weekend trip where they get to choose all of the activities (even paintball if they want). During treatment, she forewarned them that she wouldn't have her hair on and they'd have to be OK with it. Who wouldn't agree? Janet laughs with the memory, *"The five-year-old teased me at one point by saying, 'Put your wig back on; you're starting to scare me!'"*

Janet admits she even liked it when her friend's boyfriend called her *"cancer girl"*. Her parents didn't like it much, but she appreciated his casual and comfortable humor. *"I chose to go bald on camping trips with my friends. It's amazing how my guy friends opened up because of that. Now I just warn them that I can't stand too close to the flames. Since I can't feel anything, I might catch on fire. One of those same friends tells me 'I'm just happy you're here!' every New Year's Eve as he gives me a kiss.*

"I was very crabby the day I was tattooed in preparation for radiation. Tears were streaming even though it wasn't painful. I just desperately wanted to be done. I was tired, just wanted to get rid of it and move on. Someone said to me around that time, 'This must have you thinking about your mortality.' My response? 'No! This is just a bump in the road.' Yes it was a loss, but I was becoming more philosophical about it."

Once radiation was completed, Janet participated in a clinical trial for a new cancer-deterring drug, Herceptin. She was selected because she fit all of the conditions for the trial (as did a 90-year-old woman). For an entire year, she had weekly half-hour infusions of the drug. Her heart was monitored throughout to ensure that there wasn't any detrimental impact. Although it was a bit of a hassle to check in once a week, there were no side effects.

After going in twice a week to expand her skin, Janet had reconstructive surgery in May 2001. Surgery over, she rushed home to tell her roommate, *"You've got to see these!"* Due to swelling, her breasts initially looked like double D's. Janet's sister playfully agreed to make a note on her organ donation card to give Janet a nipple. In the meantime, Janet had nipples recreated and tattooed to look more natural. And the swelling did go down.

Two days after reconstruction, Janet was already anxious to get out. True to spirit, she attended a music festival with her friends. *"I tucked my drainage pouch into my pants and safety-pinned it to my shorts. It took forever to unplug everything when I had to go to the bathroom, but I didn't NOT want to be there."*

Friends and family knew the cancer card was coming whenever Janet started a sentence with, *"I have a terminal illness, so..."* Janet pulled the cancer card for such things as not wanting to run downstairs to get the milk, not wanting to sit in the back seat of the car, not wanting to organize the annual camping trip (her friends refused to accept it in that instance). To mark her one-year anniversary in December 2001, Janet gave each of her nurses a tree ornament and created a special closure gift for each family member. Along with a letter thanking each of them for their loving support and encouragement, she included a copy of the cancer card—never to be used again.

Janet's friend, who'd been diagnosed right before her, died in spring 2004. She'd urged Janet to have her ovaries removed, because she was personally convinced that her breast cancer was estrogen-related. Janet ignored her advice, but it was a very real eye-opener. *"I was honest with her. I'd avoided talking to her because it was just too close to home. I lost momentum and rolled back with her experience. I learned that I can't handle everything all of the time."*

Janet's mom watched her best friend die of breast cancer, then she had to watch her own daughter go through it. Her natural motherly response? *"I wish it had happened to me."* It's a reciprocal caring. It's hard for Janet to see that her cancer made other people sad. *"I catastrophize but try to keep it in. I've worried my mom and boyfriend enough. I'm afraid of a recurrence. I'd be devastated if I wasn't able to have children, even though I know the cancer may not be the reason behind it. I'm at a disadvantage for the future—I'm not supposed to have kids for five years. I lost crucial years of normal stuff. But then I think, whose life is normal? My story is so easy compared with other women. My world wasn't collapsing. My family and friends never left my side. I never had to worry about money or my job."*

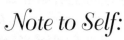

Note to Self:

It's natural to go into a downward spiral when other people die from the same disease as yours, especially if it's a friend or family member. Talk to a counselor or psychologist to help you through that double whammy.

At a recent baseball game, her brother noticed that she hadn't played her best and asked if she was upset about it. A formerly competitive Janet answered, *"Who cares? Some things aren't that big a deal anymore."* She gets greater enjoyment from just being together and having fun than from winning a game.

"I've learned a lot about myself. I don't have to be perfect. The medication has caused a weight gain, but I'm OK with that. There's a deeper, more substantive side to me now. I told myself 'You will get through this' and I thought it would be in the front of my mind forever, but sometimes I actually forget I had cancer."

For her 30th birthday party, Janet's hair had grown back and she'd planned a party, but her family surprised her with one instead. Janet thought she was headed to yet another baby shower for her new nephew who was born unexpectedly seven weeks early. What she didn't realize was that there were nearly 100 family members and friends gathered waiting to celebrate her, not the baby.

The Tamoxifen can make Janet very cranky and irritable. *"It's like PMS+. I have changed. I'm faster paced and have a lot of urgency now. I can be so impatient with people and I've been called on it at work. I just want to fix problems and move on. I have more gumption."* That gumption has led Janet to become an active volunteer and fundraiser for cancer research. She recruited seventy family members and friends for the breast cancer walk in 2003 and they held a joy-filled picnic after. People from all parts of her life, workmates, friends, family, even cousins, helped raise $4000 for the American Cancer Society. That year, Janet was the honorary cancer survivor and appeared on the local TV news.

"For Breast Cancer Awareness Month, I volunteered to hand out flyers at a large department store. I spent four hours standing next to Miss USA, a 19-year-old, size 2, who had selected breast cancer as her cause. I learned all about pageants, the evening gown selection process, and the important things she'd learned from her experience. I'm proud to say that I kept my self-esteem and humor intact even with my weight gain and post-chemo short hair. I was able to laugh when I thanked them for standing me next to the pretty girl.

"I'm not a crier, but at my six-month check-ups, I cry happy tears because I'm so ecstatic. For Thanksgiving 2003, I had a turkey party and I was so grateful just to be happy, to have a roof over my head and to have twenty-two people I loved gathered at my house."

Looking ahead, Janet is passionate about the course she has developed and will begin facilitating for the Young Survival Coalition, a support group for young women. *"Now I need to help other young women early on with the emotional issues of a cancer diagnosis."* She's spent months gathering the support and certification she needed to bring her dream to reality.

Janet is close to the four-year marker. At five years, the chance for recurrence drops to 3 to 5%. Is it surprising to know that she's already planning a huge celebratory party?

Breath-holding

Once a breast cancer patient, always a breast cancer patient. My next mammogram will mark the first anniversary of my breast cancer surgery. Since the day I received the reminder letter, I've found myself holding my breath whenever my mind wanders to that appointment and the potential outcome. No longer can I casually schedule a mammogram and erase it from my mind until it occurs. I'll never regain my former cloak of invulnerability. Not until my mind moves onto another topic do I relax enough to inhale a full, deep breath.

At my six-month post-lumpectomy, post-radiation mammogram, I didn't realize I was holding my breath until after the results were back. The mammogram was unexpectedly painful (my breast was still healing) and shallow breathing was all I could manage between pictures. I then sat alone in the room multi-tasking—breathing tentatively, reading a travel magazine, keeping my thoughts occupied, avoiding the recollection of the mammogram when my cancer first appeared, falling just short of positive-thinking—waiting for the results.

The door opened and my heart jumped as I rose from my chair. Then it jumped again to see the radiologist, the nurse clinician and my husband all enter the room together. "What the matter? What's the matter? Why are you all here?" With ears buzzing from lack of oxygen, I heard them say, "Everything's clear, everything looks good, everything's fine…" Breathing in through every bodily pore, I then heaved a sigh that dissolved into tears of relief.

Breath-holding is a common experience for breast cancer survivors. How many of us are holding our breaths in unison at any given time? Is it a stretch to believe that an unspoken prayer goes up each time a breath is held? Unknown to each of us, the woman sitting next to us might be sending up her own silent, breathless prayer along with our own.

—Christy L. Schwan

Jenell, age 43

*A*s she gazes at her reflection in the mirror, my hand instinctively reaches out to rub her round, balding head, and we smile poignantly at each other. It is the first time I've seen her without the wig and I'm touched that she felt comfortable enough to remove it. In the five years since we've seen each other, it feels like several lifetimes have passed. She picks up on that fleeting thought and comments on how many lifetimes we actually experience during this one lifetime. When we're deep in the middle of one of our lifetimes, it seems to go on forever and then once we're through it, it seems like someone else's life we dreamed.

That's the wonder of our relationship. An embryonic thought passes between us and is nurtured and birthed by the other. She is my muse and I hers. Our philosophical exchanges are effortless, at times rambling, often irreverent, frequently insightful, typically amusing. Our discussions end alternately with a lingering sigh or a burst of laughter.

I tell her about prior conversations that have stuck in my mind, shaped my life and made me who I am. She doesn't remember what I remember and the memories significant to her have escaped me. She's incredulous that an offhand comment she made years ago still stings with its recollection. *"You're just collecting 'yeses'"*, was her livid commentary on the job offers I'd received when I'd decided to discontinue my consulting practice and go back to Corporate America. I refuse the apology she now offers. Her insights kept me honest with myself over these past few years.

I force myself to accept the reality of her situation. I force myself to stop trying to fix her health. I force myself to let her be herself. I force myself to keep from crying. I force myself…

It's a wonder we ever met. I was introduced to her by a friend of a friend of a business acquaintance. We were both reluctant transplants to Cincinnati, making the best of it by keeping a running commentary on the idiosyncrasies of the city. Neither of us could have imagined that we'd both be initiated into the breast cancer sisterhood. We'd lost touch for several years when I moved back to Wisconsin. After my own diagnosis, I spent months searching for her and eventually tracked her down at her parent's home. So, this is Jenell's story as best as I can tell it.

The lump seemed to appear overnight. When she met with the doctor, he was immediately concerned and tests revealed a fast growing form of invasive breast cancer. Along with his recommendation that she *"Just go ahead and have a double mastectomy, since your breasts are really small anyway"*, he supplied her with medical books showing graphic pictures of women before and after surgery. A free spirit, Jenell naturally bolted. Her support system in Cincinnati encouraged her to explore alternative therapies in lieu of medical intervention. It was the thread of hope she was desperately seeking. A thread that began to unravel quickly.

*J*ust go ahead and have a double mastectomy, since your breasts are really small anyway.

Within a month of diagnosis, she began following the misguided, mind-controlling directives of a noted, but unsubstantiated, spiritual shaman. She sold her home, packed up her belongings, moved to California and traveled to Mexico for a prescription for Gerson therapy. With a *"promise"* that she would be healed within three months, she devoted herself to an intense juicing diet, herbal vitamins and supplements, coffee enemas, colonics and meditation. Cut off from her family, she became convinced that her cancer had developed because she needed a dramatic change in her life. Her dual goal at that point in time was to: 1. avoid the truth about her illness and 2. avoid unnecessary pain. She notes pensively that both have come back to her in spades.

In the twelve months that she diligently followed the instructions of her *"healer"*, the cancer metastasized to her bones. She was unaware that untreated breast cancer had the potential to move to and attack other parts of her body. By the time she finally had her mastectomy, she had lost so much weight that the surgeon could not perform reconstructive surgery because there was not enough fat left in her body to build a breast. Shortly after her mastectomy was performed, her hipbones had deteriorated to the point where she had to have an emergency hip replacement at the age of 44.

Jenell has since been in constant, unremitting pain. Her doctors have been surprised by the increase in her pain threshold as the cancer has moved through her neck and spine and only recently put her on a combination of morphine, steroids and radiation therapy. Jenell walks with a cane and has a special electronic recliner that helps her both sit and stand. On my first visit, she gave me a demonstration along with a state-fair-barker running commentary on its unique features. We laughed together at the absurdity of it all.

I believe my job is to listen, to help her over the anger hurdles that threaten to consume her, to help her find the peace and resolution and comfort she seeks.

Jenell is no saint though. She struggles to bring a perspective to the probable brevity of her life and the way it is ending. She is often overcome with anger, even hatred, towards her *"healer"*, the insensitive medical advisors with whom she originally consulted and the former friends who blithely encouraged her choices. Regrets over her own decisions eat away at her as much as the cancer does at times. I believe my job is to listen, to help her over the anger hurdles that threaten to consume her, to help her find the peace and resolution and comfort she seeks.

The Blue Tattoo Club

She may not be a saint, but she is a winsome sage, "*You know, it's really for the best that I'm experiencing my old age at 45. At least this way, I have my parents to take care of me, rather than spending my time alone at 90 in a nursing home.*" I'm initially taken aback at how casually she makes that declaration and then I can only nod my head in silent agreement. She's right. There could be no better comfort than having your own mother care for you during this stage of your life. A mother touches all of your senses with favorite foods, remembered scents, loving embraces, a familiar smile, a calming voice. She can bring an ease to any situation which no one else can.

Not that it's easy for her mother. For my monthly visits, Caroline always prepares a lovely, fine-linen-best-china luncheon, leaving Jenell and me to talk in private. She joins us for the special desserts she has fixed, making us feel like we've just been to a fancy tearoom.

In the few minutes that she and I have spent alone, Caroline expresses the anguish she feels over Jenell's condition. If only, if only, if only—she wonders if she should have forced Jenell into a different choice. But what mother has ever been able to convince her strong-willed, independent daughter (whether 4 or 44) to do something against her will? A mother carries her child's pain in her own chest. Self-forgiveness does not come easily. It's so often replaced with self-flagellation.

Strong-willed, stubborn, single-minded. Like mother, like daughter? Opposites in many ways, yet there's a genetic resonance that can't be ignored. Jenell eloquently expresses that living together as adults she is now experiencing her mother *"full throttle"*. As her own motor slows down, her mother's revs up, earnestly trying to help Jenell hold on. When does realism replace optimism? When does hope become acceptance? When does holding on loosen its grip and gently begin letting go?

Her sisters bring perpetual, yet unrealistic, optimism with them at each visit. Ever hopeful, they cling to the belief that if they can just get Jenell moving and out of the house, her health will start to improve. Their most recent goal was to take her on a day trip to the Chicago Zoo. I can hear her bemused smile over the phone as she tells me that renting a wheelchair is the least of the issues. It's a new body that she needs to rent since sitting anywhere other than in the sheltering arms of her electronic recliner causes more pain than she can handle these days.

I'm not ready to give her up quickly now that I've found her again. I ask surreptitiously when she thinks she might be able to take a trip with me to a retreat center off the coast of Seattle. She gives me a quirky, crooked smile and says, *"Christy, I'll have to come as a bird— it's the only way I'd be able to make it that far and across the sea."* And that launches us into a conversation about what type of bird she wants to be so that I can be sure to know it's her when I see it. We have not yet settled on the bird, so it somehow assures me that we have more time.

I'd wanted to resume our email reflections and had Jenell's computer repaired for that purpose. By the time I'd gotten it back to her, she no longer had the energy to either sit or compose. I resort to daily telepathy, keeping her old picture business card front and center on my office desk, so that I think of her often and send a prayer her way.

Seeking her insight, I take along several freshly written essays on one of my visits. With her energy sagging in the afternoon light, she asks me to read them to her. I hesitate, realizing that I've never read my own works out loud. I begin with a light piece about living a catless life. As I continue, she nods and says, *"uh, huh"* in agreement. She pauses reflectively when I finish and then the inherent editor takes control and she begins her critique. I listen in amusement. Welcome back, my old Jenell, even if just for a minute. She looks up and we exchange knowing smiles.

The Blue Tattoo Club

When I call, her voice is strong and she wants to spend little of our time discussing her health status. She prefers to take the interviewer role, asking about the details of my life, my family, my health, my career. There is a subtle energy exchange that occurs during our phone conversations. Is it possible that we lift each other out of our doldrums?

Nearly six months have now passed since we re-found each other. I call to schedule my monthly visit. It takes a while for Jenell to answer. When she does, her voice has changed. She's just returned from a three-week stay in the hospital, where the doctors worked to get her pain back under control. I've just returned from a family vacation in the north woods, achingly unaware of her misery. What happened to my supposed telepathic connection? How could I not know that she was suffering?

> *What happened to my supposed telepathic connection? How could I not know that she was suffering?*

Her voice has no hint of self-pity. Rather it seems filled with disbelief. She tells me that while her pain is again mercifully under control, she's now paralyzed from the chest down. Aware that the cancer had spread from her bones to her tissue, she was prepared to slip quietly into a coma once the cancer invaded her brain cells. She wasn't prepared for paralysis. She's returned home, now under hospice care, with her three sisters taking weekly turns to care for her. I have no words, other than *"I love you. When can I see you next?"* Her final words before I hang up the phone? *"This really sucks, Christy."*

So we live our lives day by day, knowing this lifetime will be over soon enough and we will move into the next. Jenell feels an advantage in knowing that she can see the end, whereas I cannot. Self-deceptive or self-assured? It's irrelevant. Jenell seems to have relaxed into a realm of calm acceptance.

I pray for her comfort. I pray for days of relief, peace and even joy. I pray for her spirit to be lifted whether through a favorite TV show (she admits she's become addicted to Crossing Over), her cat's gentle, protective cuddling, the special desserts her mother prepares for us, or the sun-dappled trees outside her window. I pray for her.

> *I pray for her comfort. I pray for days of relief, peace and even joy. I pray for her spirit to be lifted.*

There is a physics term called half-life that is used to describe how long an element will give off radiation. My hope is to live to be at least ninety. Cancer and its associated therapies have cut Jenell's life short. She may not live to see 46, but in her half-life, she has remained real and true to herself. She states emphatically that she does not want her memorial service or obituary to proclaim her a hero or to describe her valiant battle against cancer. She is not a contender for canonization (admittedly a little hard for a Lutheran to achieve) nor is she a poster child for positive thinking. Yet she is the wounded healer that her charlatan shaman predicted. The difference is that her physical wounds have not healed. Her words are the healer, her story is the healer, her life is the healer. I am just her storyteller, so that other women will know that some choices hold less promise than others.

When I was leaving from my last visit with Jenell in October, 2003, I mentioned I'd be back between Thanksgiving and Christmas. She paused, gave me one of her knowing smiles and finally said, *"Well, I'm not sure where I'm going to be then."* I responded, *"I know, Sweetie, I'll call first."* She knew that time was short and had packed as much into that visit as possible. We'd had a lengthy discussion that day about God, faith and forgiveness, life after death, believing versus knowing. Jenell stated at one point, *"Well, considering the shape I'm in, I just want to make sure I've covered all my bases!"*

Jenell had a unique ability to cover all her bases. When I first met her, I'd never known anyone who had two business cards. She had one noting her left brain capabilities as a writer, speaker and consultant, the other highlighting her right brain talents as an actress, model and spokesperson. She could make an entire room of strangers turn their heads—first with her beauty, class and style and then with a belly laugh so loud and infectious that everyone wished they were in on the joke. She was strong-willed yet sensitive, sweet yet sarcastic, confident yet conflicted. She charmed everyone she touched. She brought a richness and depth to our relationship that I've had with no other friend.

> *She charmed everyone she touched. She brought a richness and depth to our relationship that I've had with no other friend.*

Jenell left two voice mail messages for me the weekend before she died in late November 2003. Her voice was weak as she asked me to come visit one last time. I'd been out of town for the weekend. By the time I received the message and called her back, she was in and out of consciousness, unable to speak any longer. Her sister agreed to put the phone to Jenell's ear so that she could hear my voice. I reminded her of how much I loved her and the friendship we held dear. I assured her that my husband would conduct her funeral service as she had hoped he would. I could hear her keening cry and her raspy *"Thank you, thank you, thank you."* Her sister came back on the line and asked if I'd heard Jenell say she loved me, too. My heart and tears burst on hearing that. I saved those two voice mails until the following May, unable to push the delete button. They were my one last worldly connection to Jenell.

Jenell, I know you're listening today. Let me just say that God doesn't care which base you made it to, He just cares that you were in the game. I know He's wrapped his arms around you and you're both smiling your knowing smiles. I love you and you're in my heart forever.

Easy For You To Say

malignancy, biopsy
easy for you to say
how can this be happening to me?
talk to me

in situ, stage II
easy for you to say
how can this be happening to me?
talk to me

lumpectomy, mastectomy
easy for you to say
how can this be happening to me?
talk to me

oncology, chemotherapy
easy for you to say
how can this be happening to me?
talk to me

path report, med port
easy for you to say
how can this be happening to me?
talk to me

radiation, tamoxifin
easy for you to say
how can this be happening to me?
talk to me

hormone receptor, breast cancer
easy for you to say
how can this be happening to me?
talk to me

—Christy L. Schwan

Jenifer, age 46

A single parent with a twenty-five year-old son, Jenifer is a warmly vibrant, earnestly positive woman. Her smile and laugh quickly light up the room as she and her sister, Laurel, begin her story. She starts by telling me that her menstrual period had returned after nearly a year's absence and she's feeling like she's twelve years old again. Since she's 47 now, she was just fine thinking that chemotherapy had put her into premature menopause. So at first she was in denial about her period, thinking she'd accidentally scratched herself. She was totally unprepared with no supplies, other than paper towels, to handle the flow once it really started going. *"I fussed over myself all day! Although it's a good sign that my body continues to recover, not having periods was one of the positive outcomes of my treatment."*

Jenifer was diagnosed in February 2003. She does have a family history of breast cancer, including a sister, yet she hadn't had a mammogram for over three years. *"I know it was stupid, but I didn't like the way they handled my past mammogram and ultrasound. It took a long time for the radiologist to read my results. I ended up waiting alone for what seemed liked hours, while the nurse kept nervously popping in on me either saying nothing at all or making inane comments like, 'Oh good, you're reading a magazine.'"*

Jenifer had noticed the lump on a Saturday night as she was smoothing her nightgown over her body. Back and forth from breast to breast, muttering to herself *"Is there or isn't there?"* By Sunday she was finally convinced there was a lump. A quick call on Monday morning resulted in an immediate appointment. *"All you have to do is say lump and they squeeze you right in."*

Her doctor left several messages for her later that week, then gave her the initial news over the phone—the mammogram and ultrasound had confirmed a lump. Within two weeks, a needle aspiration and biopsy were completed. In early March, a lumpectomy was performed because her surgeon thought she was too young for a mastectomy. Ten lymph nodes were removed and all were clear. *"I'm in love with my doctors, nurses and surgeon who all made it so much more endurable than I could have thought. My mom spends the winters in Florida and wanted to come home to be with me during the surgery, but I told her not to come since I was in such good hands. I told her I might need her more later."*

Because everything had gone so well before and after surgery, she was very hopeful when she met with the oncologist. Expecting to be in and out within minutes, she didn't ask her son or sister to accompany her as they had on all other appointments. The appointment lasted three hours. *"It was three horrific hours of crying. I wasn't in denial. I was just so shocked*

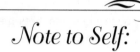

Note to Self:

Specific words can unleash an emotional hurricane. Recognizing those hot buttons can help you regain your equilibrium more quickly.

about the need for chemo. Everything had been so positive up to that point, I wasn't prepared for the recommendation. I realized that I associated chemo, not cancer, with death. Reality hit hard when the nurse handed me a hat that had been made by volunteers. When I finally got home that day, I threw that hat on a bench and refused to look at it again."

Jenifer scheduled her chemo treatments for every third Friday and planned her work as a subsidized housing specialist around them. Blood draws were done the week before and the day of each chemo. Her oncologist explained that if her white blood cell count wasn't high enough on those days, they'd have to delay the treatment.

Jenifer was adamant about sticking to her schedule so that she'd have the weekend and Monday to recover after each chemo. *"I lived on the edge each chemo day, praying for a high white blood cell count. At the same time, I dreaded the shots that were necessary to bolster my count. It's painful when your bone marrow is forced to go into overdrive* producing white blood cells. Even with pain medication, my bones and heart literally ached. But my prayers were answered. My blood count was consistently high, so I never had to waver from my plan. Most people never knew the pain and anxiety I was going through in preparation for each chemo. I wanted to be strong so that it would be easier on others.

"My mom and niece came to every chemo treatment with me, comforting and supporting me with their love and hugs. My sense of humor kept me going, but my niece became suspicious of my perpetually happy face and asked me if I was faking it. It was hard to admit that at times I just wanted people to leave, so I could be alone with my thoughts. I'm used to taking care of others, so the role reversal was uncomfortable. It's draining to see everyone else worrying and it can be overwhelming to experience love on the surface."

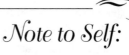

Note to Self:

Love on the surface is raw, unhidden care and concern. It's OK to need and ask for alone time, to pace yourself emotionally, to recover from that outpouring.

In preparation for the side effects of chemo, Jenifer purchased the requisite over-the-counter constipation and diarrhea medications as well as a prescription anti-nausea drug. She set up a *"cancer corner"* in her medicine chest. She and Laurel planned an extended weekend pajama party after the first chemo treatment. They religiously gave Jenifer a dose of the anti-nausea drug every 3 to 4 hours and waited for her to feel sick. When the nausea never started, they continued the dosage. By Sunday afternoon, Jenifer was still feeling great, so they agreed *"What the heck? Let's go shopping!"* They later learned they'd been overdosing her on the anti-nausea medication.

In retrospect, Laurel mentions that an aunt of theirs had died of bone cancer a decade earlier. Although they hadn't seen her after the start of chemo, they'd heard that she had literally crawled from her car to her kitchen floor after each treatment. They promised each other to do everything they could to keep that from happening to Jenifer.

Jenifer kept misplacing her bottle of anti-nausea meds and even though it was expensive, she'd have to get another refill before each chemo. It wasn't until after chemo was over that she found all those missing bottles in the opposite corner of her medicine cabinet. She chalks it up to chemo-brain.

Jenifer expected to lose her hair by Easter but she vowed that she'd never wear a turban. Laurel recalls that Jenifer brought along a baggie of hair clippings to her hair appointment several weeks before. Not wanting to say the wrong thing or discourage her, Laurel silently wondered if Jenifer expected the hairdresser to somehow reattach the strands (perhaps with two-way tape). Says Laurel, *"We all got a good laugh out of my absurd notion, when I realized that the hairdresser was going to use the clippings to find the right color and texture match for Jenifer's wig."*

Note to Self:

Jenifer's support group held activities such as "beaded bracelet time" as a way to lighten the tough conversations. If you're inclined to group meetings, find a group with a comforting atmosphere, where questions can be asked freely and answers are not too clinical.

A true friend, the hairdresser came to Jenifer's home on Good Friday. *"There were never any clumps on my pillow, but when my hair began following my brush that morning, I called and she came over immediately with a bottle of wine. She shaved my head in the garage, where there were no mirrors and she did not let one strand of hair fall in my view. When she finished, she told me that I had a beautifully shaped head. I went into hibernation the rest of the weekend. On Monday morning, I just smiled and kept on walking when my co-workers complimented my cute, new haircut. Laurel liked the style of my wig so much, she went out and got a matching haircut!*

"Losing my hair was the biggest realization that the chemo was going to put my body through significant change. I kept telling myself that the poison was going to help, but it's hard not knowing what the

outcome is going to be. The possibility of breast cancer is part of being a woman and there's nothing I can do to change that. I've always talked to God. I see His hand in my life and I get hope and strength from that."

While the blonde is from a bottle, Jenifer's hair has grown back curly. *"It's amazing how cold the top of your head can get. I don't know how bald guys can handle it. I developed this little ritual of pulling my blankets up on both sides of my ears to keep them warm and still find myself doing that when I'm cold."*

During chemo, Jenifer detected a noticeable urine scent that seemed to seep from every pore in her body. Hesitant to mention it to anyone, she privately asked her support group nurse, who in turn suggested she bring it up at the following meeting. With a sigh of relief, several other women acknowledged they'd experienced the same odor, although undetectable to anyone else.

After a half-dozen bruises from failed attempts at locating a viable vein for chemo, a port was inserted in her chest after the second chemo treatment. The round, quarter-sized box is inserted just under the skin and is covered by a thin membrane. It's a lingering reminder of chemo, since the port must be left in for a year following treatment and must be flushed out every four weeks to avoid infection. *"I felt like the Bride of Frankenstein with the port and the tube up my neck. I set off the metal detectors in Target more than once, so I made sure to keep my medical alert ID card handy. I often thought it would be great to have an inspirational message on the back of the medical alert I.D. cards. A simple reminder to keep things in perspective."*

While it wasn't easy to ask, Jenifer found that even casual acquaintances were willing to help. Her most vivid memory is running out of constipation tablets during one of her chemo weekends. Without hesitation, her next door neighbor ran to the drugstore and then quietly left them outside her door so as not to disturb her.

Jenifer is an avid movie lover and indulged herself by renting multiple videos during her chemo weekends. On one particularly rough weekend, she asked the video store manager to charge her up front for an extra day since she knew wouldn't be able to return it on time. He generously waived the extra fee when he found out the reason for the request. Jenifer's memories of these simple acts of kindness linger long after the treatments have ended.

"I was a little disappointed that some of the people at work were curious, but seemed too afraid to ask. When people were tiptoeing around after I returned from surgery, I pulled aside my jacket and said, 'Look, I have half a boob now, OK?' I must have done that at least half a dozen times until other people were comfortable that I was comfortable talking about it.

"One thing I loved about my male friends and brother-in-law is that they did ask a lot of questions. The biggest jokester at my office offered to drive me to appointments and frequently checked to see if I needed anything. When my flippant response was 'I'm fine!', he'd stop me cold by asking, 'NO! Are you REALLY OK?' Those bursts of love gave me back more than I ever lost."

Jenifer's niece gave her a picture book entitled *The Meaning of Life* by Bradley Trevor Greive. This little book, with a big green frog on the front, was inspirational and uplifting for Jenifer. The gentle humor and insight gave her a comforting perspective.

With the last day of chemo scheduled near her birthday, Jenifer's co-workers planned a celebration barbeque. *"It was heaven! The support and love and rejoicing were incredible. My mother was there just as she had been for every one of my chemo treatments. This was a major stepping stone for me—I'd made it through my chemo without losing myself."*

> ### Note to Self:
> Gratitude… A big deal to you may be a little deal to me and vice versa. Be grateful for both the big and little.

Six weeks of radiation therapy quickly followed the celebration. Jenifer was barely able to keep her eyes open on the drive home after the treatments. She developed shingles around her waistline and her resistance fell so low that the doctors threatened to quarantine her. In response, her co-workers sprang into protective action. They kept unhealthy residents away from her, sniffles weren't allowed and a can of Lysol was perpetually in use. The quarantine was never imposed.

Despite her fatigue, Jenifer set a personal goal of getting her radiation therapist to talk to her. Jenifer had early on given her the nickname "Lurch" since she rarely spoke and primarily communicated through hand gestures. Unsuccessful until the final treatment, Jenifer dropped her hospital gown to reveal the upside down smiley face she'd drawn on her own chest. Lurch burst out laughing with *"Take care, I hope all goes well!"* Jenifer achieved two milestones that day and thankfully the hardest part was washing off the magic marker.

Jenifer and her son are very close and affectionate, yet she was always careful to keep her hat on when he came to visit. He called her recently at 1:30 a.m. after watching the movie Calendar Girls to say, *"The cancer didn't really hit me until now. I just need to tell you how much I love you, Mom."*

With successful treatment behind her, Jenifer has one standing request of her sister, Laurel. *"My son is an only child of a single mom. If in the future something were to happen to me, I need you to be his Mom—his real mom. A mom that will tell him if he's being a jerk, if he's going in the wrong direction, to keep him connected to the rest of the family. Don't lose him, don't let him go."* Laurel has agreed to be that mom.

Jenifer continues to gain perspective and insight from her support group where a new member is keeping everyone laughing with her cancer commentary. The Arimidex that Jenifer will take for the next five years has caused her to gain some weight, but nothing can hide her smile, her joy, her hope.

Radiation Girl

On the first day of my radiation therapy, my grown son called to see how I was doing and he asked to talk to Radiation Girl. At my laughing response, we both imperceptibly recalibrated our emotional gauges regarding breast cancer, realizing that:

- *I can still laugh.*
- *He can still make me laugh.*
- *His status as family comedian remains intact.*
- *Cancer isn't so serious that it can't be made fun of.*
- *Any discomfort from radiation therapy can be ignored, at least temporarily.*

I have to admit, my new title conjured up a brief vision of a glowing caped crusader flying by. I don't recall the color of the cape, whether pastel or a vivid primary color. But I do remember thinking it was a pretty powerful image. From my comic book reading days, I remember that most super heroes came by their powers through some mystical interaction with energy, either nuclear or electrical.

Laying in the preformed curves of the body mold, day after day, for my three minutes of radiation, I never felt heroic, just exposed. After a few weeks, I became accustomed to quickly dropping my gown while chatting with the therapists as they aligned my tattoos with the direction of the beams. They would scurry out of the room and communicate via intercom. I'd lay there wondering at the power of the technology as it buzzed its way toward any remaining cancer cells. I'd counted down the days using fractions as my markers—1/7, 1/5, 2/7, 2/5, 3/7, 1/2 of the way through.

This week marks an even greater triumph—the one-year anniversary of the end of my radiation treatment. Semi-annual mammograms indicate that I am cancer-free. Maybe my son was right. Where's my cape? I do feel like I can fly!

—*Christy L. Schwan*

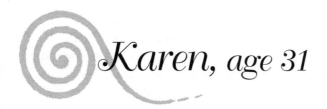

Karen, *age 31*

*K*aren is an avid gardener wannabe, reader, home decorator, and shopaholic who loves a good party. She's also an enthusiastic and beloved 4th grade schoolteacher, who has extreme patience with her students, but outside the classroom she can't even wait for the calendar to change. She has a tendency to be obsessive/compulsive about keeping things neat and clean. Even though she's the youngest of four girls, she likes to be in charge and loves to help her sisters with their decorating. Light-hearted yet quick-tempered, blunt but caring, Karen is the family peace keeper. She met her husband at fifteen even though they didn't marry until their mid-20s. Their daughter was just nine months old when Karen's cancer diagnosis was made.

She had limited success breastfeeding her daughter, who tended to favor Karen's left breast, so after three months she switched to formula. Then in December 1998, Karen noticed that her nipples were secreting colostrum liquid. Her sister, a practicing nurse, said to contact her OB/GYN. Her mother assured her that she'd be fine, even though Karen's grandmother had noticed a lump while she'd been breastfeeding Karen's mom decades before. Her grandmother had waited ten years before finally having a mastectomy and died when Karen was just a baby.

Everyone had said not to worry, so her husband had taken their daughter in for her six-month pictures while Karen had gone to the appointment alone. The nurse felt a mass on Karen's right side. After the first mammogram of her life, Karen was told they needed another film on the left and an ultrasound on the right. *"It was surreal. There I was lying on my back while the same technician who'd done my pregnancy ultrasound a year earlier was now checking for cancer. Nothing was found on the right side, but my heart sank when the radiologist wanted to talk. 'You'll want to make a bee line out the door as soon as I say this.' He was concerned about an area of calcifications in my left breast, so they dialed the number of my OB/GYN for me. My OB/GYN told me to call a specific surgeon to make an appointment for a biopsy to be done immediately. I was shaking so hard that I could barely drive home. I'll never forget the picture of my husband standing, my daughter eating and my niece coloring as I walked in the door of my house and fell to the ground sobbing."*

On December 23rd, Karen's husband went to the hospital with her for the stereotactic biopsy. *"I remember thinking, 'What am I doing here? I just delivered my baby.' And I was still curious about my right breast as my left breast was hanging down during the procedure. They told me the results would be ready in two days—my daughter's first Christmas.*

"I memorized every detail of the elaborate Christmas dinner my sister cooked for the family that year. The dining table was set up in our gorgeous, decorated-just-like-homes-in-the-Christmas-section-of-the-newspaper living room, in front of a huge crackling fire. It was a wonderful Christmas. Yet I looked at my daughter in her red velvet dress and I couldn't help thinking 'This may be my last Christmas ever.'"

Wait, wait, wait. Karen was watching the news, holding her daughter in her arms when the call came at 5:15 p.m. on December 28th. *"It* didn't come back in our favor Karen. You have cancer." Her husband caught the baby as Karen dropped her. *"All I heard was 'Call Dr. Vincent', then just 'wanh, wanh, wanh' like the voices of the off-screen parents in a Charlie Brown cartoon. I wanted to scream, 'Just stop talking and let me hang up!' It was the first time I'd seen my husband cry."*

Karen's greatest fear was that her daughter would grow up without a mother. Sad, numb, and scared, she vowed to keep a journal for her daughter (a journal that detailed her walk with cancer, but more importantly, captured the memories of her daughter's babyhood, memories that Karen was afraid her husband wouldn't remember).

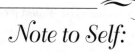

Note to Self:

Women are the memory keepers. Journaling has a dual benefit as a healing catharsis and a recollection tool.

Karen's initial journal entry says: *I didn't think of death. I thought of you, your dad and myself. How were we going to get through this? What the hell was going to happen to me? I denied it all. I still do. It was awful. I fell to the floor in sobs. I couldn't breathe. I cried and cried. You had woken up and cried too—screamed actually.*

Karen called her parents and asked both of them to get on the line. She knew her mom would be worried because she'd cared for her own mother. Only two words came out, *"It's cancer."* Her mother's instant response? *"It's going to be OK."*

Karen's parents and husband went with her to meet the surgeon who recommended a mastectomy of the left breast, followed by chemo and radiation. He also wanted to perform an open biopsy on the right side. As the details of her family's medical history were recorded, Karen was shocked and embarrassed when her mother admitted that she'd never had a mammogram. *"I was scared shitless. It felt like I was sitting back in a recliner and letting everyone do things for me, making and helping me make decisions."*

Finally good news! The mass on the right side turned out to be an infection from breastfeeding; otherwise, Karen would have needed a double mastectomy. *"Thank goodness for my daughter. If I hadn't breastfed and developed the infection, I wouldn't have known I had breast cancer until much later."*

In the meantime, Karen met with the plastic surgeon to begin preparation for reconstruction. Karen describes him as a phenomenal man who always made her feel beautiful. He was the best at his craft, had a wonderful bedside manner and worked in tandem with the surgeon. They planned a mastectomy with a TRAM FLAP, repositioning her navel and giving her a tummy tuck in the process. Karen thought she had a lot of fat to offer since she'd just had a baby, so she tried to wheedle a little bit more out of him, *"Can't you take some off the ass, too, or at least throw in a little liposuction?"* He assured her that there was enough skin and fat from her stomach area alone.

But the reality still hit Karen hard. *"I'm a girl. What am I going to look like? My hair, my clothes, my jewelry!"* She'd rip up the Victoria Secret catalogues when they arrived. *"Look at those beautiful women. I hate them. Why did God choose me? What was He thinking? I got angry with Him and everyone. I was only 31. The best time of my life was now torture."*

Finances also became an issue for the family. Karen had used her paid time off for maternity leave and her anxiety level increased. That weight was lifted when her fellow teachers donated 300 hours of sick leave. By the time she learned of their gift, her friend, Rhonda, had already sent thank-you cards to the donators. Karen didn't keep her cancer hidden from her students either. *"They were my kids—I had to include them. They surprised me with a We Will Miss You bulletin board with each of their names written on a pink flower."*

With mastectomy scheduled for January 23, Karen exploded when she learned that she'd be sharing a room with a very sick, elderly woman. *"Not me! You can find me a private room. My daughter will be* in here, my posse, my entourage, my group. I was firm and demanding. They ended up giving me a huge honking room! Then I hated my nurse. She wore squeaky shoes, white nylons, a skirt and nurse's cap—I called her Nurse Cratchit. I'm the former peacekeeper who turned into a real bitch.

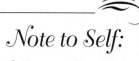

"I cope by always thinking the worst. That way I'll either be prepared or relieved. Going into surgery I told myself, 'Be strong. You will come out a totally different woman.'"

Her January 30th journal entry: *Dear Claudia, I wished to write to you but I can't believe the pain I'm in. I will explain everything that happened. I am very tired though. Going into surgery last Saturday was very scary. I remember the mask going over me and I was out. Papa, Grandma and Grandpa were there. Auntie Kathy was watching you. Anyways, I woke up in the ICU. My nurse was Elanna, such an excellent nurse! I was there for 25 hours. I was hooked up to 7 bags on my IV, heart monitor, oxygen and whatever else. I don't really remember much. I had a morphine epidural for 2+ days. It began to hurt my back. Dr. Doyle took it out Monday. I felt much better. I was so itchy all over. I didn't eat much. In the ICU all I could have was ice. I was so thirsty!! I was scared yet I knew I couldn't do anything… Thursday PM I found out (finally) that yes, the cancer is in my lymph nodes. 18 were pulled, 3 tested positive. I cried so hard. It hurts to cry. I hate it. I am so sad. I really still haven't accepted it. I watch TV and see all these women my age. I look at them and wish I was someone else.*

Young and strong, Karen's physical wounds healed very quickly and she went back to work five weeks after surgery. *"I developed a split personality: I-feel-awesome-let's-kick-ass on the outside; I'm-melting on the inside."* Karen attended only one support group meeting. As the youngest person there, she walked away feeling like no one understood her.

Her older sister, Barb, was one of her caregivers for the first six months, so they went wig shopping before chemo started. *"I'm so vain. A wig meant that the whole world would know I had cancer. As I walked in the door, the saleslady took one look at me and said, 'You look like you need a glass of wine.' I responded with, 'You're awesome! I need the whole bottle!' Instead of traumatic, it was hilarious. I'd always wanted to be a blonde, so I tried a number of fluffy blonde wigs but opted for brunette. My husband agreed that I should buy any one I wanted, since I'd be wearing it for six months."* A costume maker for the local repertory theatre highlighted and thinned out her wig to look prettier and more natural.

Karen's sister, Patty, and her mother came for her first chemo session in mid-February. She would have eight treatments, one every three weeks, followed by six weeks of radiation. Her journal entry: *Dear Claudia, Chemo started today. I'm actually having a good hair day! I picked up 'the wig'. I look like a brunette Joan Lunden. I'm afraid you might pull it off when you tug on my hair. Outside I look strong, but inside I'm not. I don't want you to be mommy-less. Wish me luck.*

The large chemo waiting room had hideous green, fake-leather, plastic covered recliners lining the walls. *"Boring, boring, boring. Every three weeks, I'd come in with my sister, Kathy, for our chemo party. We'd rearrange the room, bring in our own videos and feast the entire time. Nothing tasted good, but my sister indulged me with incredible*

> ## Note to Self:
> Rearrange whatever you need to make yourself more comfortable: your schedule, your food, your videos, your furniture, your waiting room, your life.

cheesecake, so I'd eat like a horse." Karen scheduled chemo on Fridays so she could more easily take the day off, recover over the weekend and then get back to her normal routine by Monday. Karen rewarded herself by squeezing in a quick shopping trip after each treatment.

Karen's husband, sister and her sister's boyfriend gathered together when it was time to shave her head. Ultimately, it was a relief that made her feel so much better. That summer was blistering hot. Karen never wore her wig or a hat in the house. One day she'd been outside briefly when she suddenly saw the two little boys next door come around the corner. *"I dropped to the ground. I didn't want to scare them with my bald head."* Eventually, Karen reached the point where she felt comfortable showing her college friends her bald head. They were not comfortable, but she still wanted them to see what she'd gone through. Karen's leg hair continued to grow but she did have to draw on eyebrows after they fell out. She debated getting a pair of little glasses to cover her eyebrows but soon became proficient at penciling them in.

To prevent mouth sores, Karen washed her mouth out with baking soda and water daily, but her nose and mouth and gums still hurt badly. Her last four treatments were with the drug Taxol, which caused gruesome leg pains. She began popping Vicodin steadily. She asked her pastor whether she could demand God to get the cancer out of her body. His firm response? *"Yes!"* Karen was ecstatic when her period restarted in the middle of chemo. It was the sign she needed that her body was responding.

Between treatments, Karen's white blood count dropped so low that she needed Neupogen injections everyday for twenty-one days. *"The shots hurt like hell. I'd sit on the edge of the tub in the bathroom, biting on a towel, rocking back and forth until I had the courage to go through with the nightly shot. Then I'd tell my husband I was ready and he'd inject the drug into my arm. I finally asked my doctor if it could be injected into my stomach, which was already numb due to the TRAM FLAP. When the answer was yes, I wished I'd asked sooner."*

> *Note to Self:*
>
> *If you're experiencing any significant pain, don't wait to ask about or check out other alternatives. Massage, injections in a less sensitive area, drugs, even acupuncture can relieve the pain.*

Karen rewarded herself with a full-body massage the day before her last chemo treatment. She was not only free of leg pain that day, she felt like she could do cartwheels. She attributes the massage for making her final chemo painless, *"I should have had a massage every week."*

Radiation was not a big deal for Karen. She scheduled her treatments for 7:30 a.m. so that she'd be teaching by 8:30 a.m., only a half hour late. As her hair started to grow back, she knew her ride was almost over. Karen viewed the treatments as a quiet, peaceful, therapeutic resting time. She laughed with the nurses even though lifting her left arm was painful due to the removal of lymph nodes.

By the end of October, Karen's hair had grown back just enough that she decided to put aside her wig while handing out Halloween candy. *"Chemo was over. Our daughter was dressed up like a fairy. And we were sitting on the porch together waiting for the trick or treaters. Who comes by, but the Channel 12 ten o'clock news team! What a way to come out!"*

Chemo was over. Our daughter was dressed up like a fairy. And we were sitting on the porch together waiting for the trick or treaters. Who comes by, but the Channel 12 ten o'clock news team! What a way to come out!

Karen keeps the wig in a drawer as proof, maybe even as a trophy, of what she's gone through. Sometimes when she opens the drawer, she forgets it's there and thinks it's a big rat; an apt analogy in many ways.

Cancer changed Karen's life plan of having a second child. She's explained the reason to her now six-year-old daughter through a journal entry on February 4th, 1999: *I am so sad. I can't control myself. I wanted another baby so much. Tamoxifen could put me into menopause or even cause infertility. I am so sorry! I wanted you to have a brother or sister so bad!! I can't help but cry. It's so unfair to you. I know you'll grow up without siblings. It makes me so sick. Even if we could get pregnant, I don't think I could handle getting pregnant at 37 or 38 years old. It's more dangerous then. Plus, I would be terrified I'd get cancer again due to hormonal change. I feel awful. I'm so sorry.*

The Blue Tattoo Club

Karen was inundated with homemade gifts and food from her mother's well meaning co-workers, most of whom Karen didn't know. *"I know it sounds thankless, but that was a negative experience for me. It was a perpetual reminder of my breast cancer. Someone even gave*

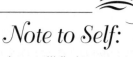

me $30 because she didn't know what else to do. I'd say thank you and then silently wish they'd just go away. I was only 31. It was overwhelming, just too much for me.

"I kept caring about how I looked, but I never really took care of my emotional well-being. My mood swings were extreme. I just wanted to go into a cocoon. I was burned and burned out after radiation. I felt like I'd had several breakdowns throughout the process and all I could do was complain, complain, complain. My husband was working so much, my baby was so needy and I was so drained. My husband is a quiet, shy, good, clean guy. He keeps me safe. My emotions were flying around and I'd worry, 'Is he sick of me? I'm so ugly.' The fear doesn't leave. I'm scared all of the time, physically and emotionally. Three months after treatment ended, I was still crying. As the days went by, I got more scared, not less. I lost a loved one—me. Acceptance and denial are still simultaneously part of me.

"I wasn't a hugely religious person, so I'd never had a true relationship with my pastor. After surgery, I remember thinking, 'Oh my God, my pastor is here. Am I dying?'" Even though she started crying every time she saw her name in the church bulletin, the perpetual reminder slowly turned into a continual confirmation that she was loved. Cancer ultimately strengthened Karen's faith and inner spirituality.

"I'm more comfortable with my body now. I still ignore the lingerie section of Victoria's Secret, but I do wear a black bikini that covers my scars. I look pretty good if you don't look at my ass, which should have been fixed by my plastic surgeon! I'm more patient with myself.

When my body is screaming, I know I need to listen. I gained a lot of weight during and after chemo. I rewarded myself by losing thirty-seven pounds through Weight Watchers and leading a healthier lifestyle. I have breasts which are finally the same size and my tummy tuck looks great. I'm waiting for the technique to be perfected before I have my nipples tattooed, so I'm not quite 'done' yet. But at the five-year mark, I look better than I did when I was diagnosed.

"I now feel very lucky that my cancer was discovered when it was. The federal law had just changed so that reconstruction after breast cancer was a covered benefit. Even though I never met her, I believe that my grandmother has been my guardian angel. My relationship with my sisters is even closer than it was before. I'm thankful to be alive, to have a fabulous family and to also have great insurance.

"A new me is finally blossoming. I'm feeling more confident and sexier. I'm clearer about who I am and what I want. I'm proud to be one of the women in this book. I'm proud of what I've gone through. I'm stronger than many women my age and feel like I can do anything. I do believe that things happen for a reason—that paths cross for a reason. I hope my story will help other women."

Less than a week after our interview, Karen's family surprised her with a Five Year Cancer-Free Party. *"My sister, Kathy, who babied me during chemo was continuing to baby me. She threw a gorgeous pink party that she'd planned for months. Pretty invitations were sent out, tulle was strung from the trees, pink lanterns and white tablecloths and chairs filled my backyard. All my close friends and family were there. My sister went above and beyond for the theme of this party. It was another step for me. It made me once again realize that what I've gone through was huge and I've survived, even when I had doubts in my mind. It was so emotional. I cried as I hugged everyone. It was a night I'll never forget. My daughter called it the "Pink Breast Cancer Party." At six, she is just beginning to understand. I hope and pray to be able to explain it to her totally one day."*

Dance Steps

Breast cancer forces women to dance a new dance. The rhythm is foreign to us. The steps can't be taught. No one else's experience can mirror our own. We stumble along, bumping into things, stubbing our toes, learning more about ourselves with each step and misstep.

Some of us do the back step willingly, even gratefully, allowing others to take the lead, be it a doctor, a family member or a friend. We defer to the experts, let others take care of us, accept advice, comply with recommendations. Now and then, even the most controlling of us slip the reins into another's hands.

Some women choose the side step, ignoring symptoms, evading tests, avoiding decisions, shutting other people out. Denial provides a momentary, much needed reprieve when we're overwhelmed by the diagnosis. Equilibrium regained, delays can gently lead us into reality.

Some of us do the two step, methodically researching, scouring the Internet, gathering all the data, exploring every alternative, polling others for their opinion. Information gathered, we armor ourselves with articles and statistics, ready to slay the dragon within.

Some women perform an erratic choreography, overloading on information, then delaying action, then going back to the experts, then second-guessing, then constricting, then pulling others close, then taking charge. We twirl and dip, dizzied by the process.

After decisions are made, after chosen treatments are completed, we're finally able to see that we've danced ourselves down a new life path. The back steps and side steps, the twirls and dips have flexed our spiritual and emotional muscles, strengthening us for our next leap—a leap we might not have had the courage or confidence to take otherwise.

—*Christy L. Schwan*

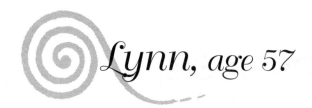

Lynn, age 57

A spiritually centered massage therapist, long-divorced mother of two adult children, grandmother to a two-year-old, Lynn has a calming voice, soothing hands, and an exploring spirit all wrapped in positive energy and quiet courage. At the age of 58, when many people are planning for retirement, Lynn started up a local Curves® fitness center whose membership has swelled to four hundred members in less than three years.

Growing up in a small town with upper class yet alcoholic parents, Lynn's earliest dreams were of getting away, finding someone else to take care of her and having a serene life. *"I spent my four years of high school in an all-girls' boarding school. My grades were Bs earned with hard work, as I now know that I'm dyslexic. I turned to sports where I was able to excel without as much frustration. We didn't have roommates, so it was a very lonely and long four years, but better than home."* Lynn's self-perception (responsible, honest, independent, stubborn, accepting and strong) was forged during this period of her life.

Four months after her regular mammogram, Lynn noticed a lump. *"I couldn't believe it since a friend of mine also discovered hers the same way. She didn't survive. I waited 3 months before going in—my daughter's wedding was coming up and I didn't want to cast a shadow on that, but the lump kept nagging me."* Notations on previous mammograms had indicated changes due to the normal aging process, but no abnormalities had been mentioned to her.

Lynn has no family history of breast cancer. But she has smoked most of her life and other family members have been struck with other forms of cancer. *"I'd received an intuitive warning about two years before my diagnosis. My response had been "No!" when I was asked if I was afraid of the Big C. I'd had some previous testing for cervical cancer, but I wasn't living in fear. I was taking nutritional supplements to keep my immune system up, though."*

When the ultrasound technician's eyes grew wide during her exam, Lynn prepared herself for the worst. The tumor was 4$^1/_2$ centimeters, putting her in the Stage 3 category. Lynn had no choice but tell her daughter who had just returned from her wedding gown fitting. *"All I could say was 'I'm sorry, I'm sorry, I'm so sorry,' between my tears. Was I afraid of the Big C now? Yes.*

"The only thing I feared at the time was ruining my daughter's wedding, but I was in great shape by then. Even with a poor prognosis, I knew it would be years before any end would come. The hardest thing for me to do was tell my family and friends without crying. I had the irrational belief that I had failed them somehow. I think I still feel that way.

"The first step I took after being diagnosed was to ask for prayers from our church and from anyone else I knew. I cried the first night then turned it over, since I'm in God's hands one way or the other. I was awed by the cards and flowers that arrived. My surgery was scheduled just two weeks before my daughter's wedding, so my friends came over and spent the day cleaning the house for me. One of my best friends took me to the doctor's from beginning to end, sharing in the initial prognosis and shock all the way through the final stitches being removed. Her presence was a great help and comfort, since I live alone and my family does not live close by. We also laughed a lot. Human behavior can be so entertaining."

Lynn chose a mastectomy since the tumor was large and she felt that not much of her breast would be left anyway if only a lumpectomy were done. A sentinel node biopsy came back clean, as was the tissue around the tumor. Six weeks had

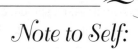

Note to Self:

We may not remember the words, we'll always remember another's presence.

elapsed from her first appointment until her surgery in mid-August, 2001. *"The night before surgery, my daughter spent the night and we took a long, midnight walk. While I don't remember the specifics of our conversation, it was a bittersweet time for both of us."*

Very little muscle tissue was removed, so Lynn needed minimal pain medication after surgery and her physical recovery was quick. The physical therapist started Lynn on flexibility and stretching exercises the day after surgery. In hindsight, she wishes she'd waited a couple of days to begin them. It would have been much less painful with little impact on her full recovery. She did experience one technical difficulty during the wedding reception—her niece's husband grabbed her for a fast dance and when he started to raise her arm to twirl her around, she had to shout, *"Wait, I can't do that yet!*

"Chemo was recommended after surgery, but after watching my friend suffer, I decided to do my own research and reading before I made a decision. I found that chemo would only increase my chance of survival by about 10%, which seemed minimal to me considering the side effects. Since there was no guarantee that chemo would cure me, I decided against it. My young doctor was stunned, but although leery, my family and friends supported my decision. No one tried to talk me out of it. I was surprised and especially pleased that my daughter accepted it."

From that point forward, Lynn launched into numerous holistic therapies including: parasitic cleansing, heat (she installed a sauna in her massage room), acupuncture, essiac herbal tea, mushroom and other nutritional supplements. From a monetary perspective, she notes that she probably spent an amount equal to what would have been her share of the co-insurance for chemo. She appealed to her insurance carrier to cover the alternative therapy because of the cost savings versus chemo, but her appeal was denied.

> ## Note to Self:
>
> *It never hurts to ask. While most alternative therapies are not covered by health insurance, the worst they can say is NO.*

Lynn attended breast cancer support group meetings only three or four times. She met several wonderful women, all of whom had gone through chemotherapy, but Lynn's choices and experiences were very different than theirs. Ultimately, the connection wasn't there for her and she stopped attending.

"People have asked me about why I didn't have chemo. Was it the loss of hair? Hardly! There are some great wigs out there these days. Though I hate to admit it, other than the side effects, my biggest concerns were: who would drive me back and forth; who would look after me if the chemo made me deathly ill; how would I continue to support myself as a massage therapist? My logical approach to declining chemo was based on my financial situation. My massage therapy practice was already shrinking since several of my long-time clients had moved out of state. Curves® became a priority for me and alternative therapies didn't deplete my energy, so I was able to keep on track with the opening date. I figured that chemo could always be my fall-back position if the holistic approach failed."

Lynn has not elected breast reconstruction. *"Perhaps if I were younger or dating, I might consider it. But my scar looks pretty good, as far as that goes. I don't even wear a prosthesis unless I'm getting dressed up. I realize it may bother some people, but I've become very comfortable with my body. If I analyze it, I want to send a message that it's OK. You don't have to have two breasts, or any, for that matter. You don't have to be ashamed of your shape, no matter what shape you're in. As I was going through some old pictures recently, I realized how great I looked when I was younger. But at the time of the photos, I only noticed my flaws and shortcomings. Are we ever 'in the present' when it comes to our own attractiveness and body image? I've always admired women who are comfortable with their size and shape. That's the subtle message I'm trying to convey.*

"Although my daughter cried when I showed her my scar, it's comforting for me to stroke it as I give thanks for my ongoing health. Checking for lumps is also a part of my daily ritual."

Lynn didn't take any fancy trips or buy herself any furs or jewelry after surgery. The Curves® start-up was Lynn's dream and it's how she rewarded herself. While she'd always been self-employed, she'd never run a business before. Life

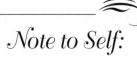

Note to Self:

Use cancer as a life liberator. Unleash your dreams.

was too short to let this challenge and opportunity pass. She certainly wasn't going to let breast cancer stand in her way. It was more than a career change. It was a life choice that gave her a focus and an avenue to bring a holistic approach to health and fitness. Her doors officially opened in November 2001.

Along with a friend who's had a kidney transplant, Lynn attended three healing services at the Basilica in downtown Chicago. Lynn experienced comfort and renewal during the *"laying on of hands"* ritual. When she was denied communion at the third service, she stopped attending but laughingly comments *"Since three is the number of completion, I felt as though I'd already received the blessing and benefit I needed."*

Lynn has her blood tested every six months and after four years she is still cancer free. Her doctor is always very pleased, relieved and somewhat surprised to see how she's coming along. *"I'm proud that I did my homework, formed my own opinions and followed through. Even though I've been alone most of my life, I've often let others influence me and my decisions, sometimes for the better, sometimes for the worse. This decision was all mine.*

"At times I'm ashamed at the lack of compassion I've felt for others in the past. I've realized that once people know what you need, more often than not, they will come through. God has been my biggest source of strength. I don't ask, 'What is the meaning of life?' or 'Why me?' It just is. Some of it I like, some of it I don't much, but it's always a challenge. Maybe I got a B+ this time. I'll find out soon enough!"

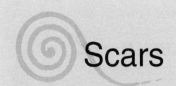# Scars

What is it that compels us to show other women our breast cancer surgery scars? Naturally, our husbands or significant others will see them. Their initial reactions are certainly important to our self-image. But there is something deeper, multi-layered about showing our scars to another woman, be it mother, daughter, sister or friend.

I've heard that some women casually lift their shirts to any and all during support group gatherings to demystify and dispel any sense of disfiguration. It's sort of like mardi gras without the beads. I applaud their bravado.

But I think back to the Christmas Eve, one week after my surgery, when I was getting dressed for the church service. My daughter didn't hesitate when I asked her if she wanted to see my scars. On the surface I'm sure I appeared casual, but once the question was out, I nearly withdrew the offer. Was it a test? Hers or mine? What response was I looking for? From her? From myself?

Only in hindsight am I able to unravel the complexity of my intent. I wanted her to understand the realness of my pain, but I didn't want her to feel sorry for me. I wanted her confirmation that I looked different, but not horrible. I wanted another female's perspective, but not judgment. I wanted her to respond honestly, but without hesitation or carefully crafted politeness. Not a simple test for anyone. Her unflinching response on viewing them, quelled my fears. "Well, if Playboy ever asks you to pose, they're going to have to do some air-brushing."

A week later, visiting my parents, my mother carefully asked if I would show her my scars. I was able to lift my shirt casually. We both agreed that they weren't too bad at all.

—*Christy L. Schwan*

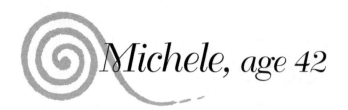

Michele, *age 42*

We met at a breast cancer support group meeting, both of us attending for the first time. I was invited to speak about the book I was working on. Michele was there at the urging of a librarian friend that had recently died of breast cancer. Michele was the life of the party, regaling her new acquaintances with one humorous, personal cancer-related anecdote after another. After she warmed up the audience, her voice suddenly broke as she described her personal journey—a journey that had begun 2 years before in mid 2001. She'd made it through her treatments with a positive, *"I will do this"* attitude, but now was angry, mad, even furious.

Michele had been experiencing swollen glands, fevers and a rash for several months prior to her diagnosis of inflammatory breast cancer, a rare and highly aggressive form of breast cancer. Inflammatory cancer accounts for only about 2% of all diagnosed breast cancers, usually affecting younger women.

Once diagnosed, Michele craved information about the disease but ruefully admits that the Internet was her downfall. *"There's way too much information out there on breast cancer that is not updated with the results of current therapies."* The initial statistics she found stated that 60% of women with inflammatory breast cancer died within five years of diagnosis. The chat rooms she visited the first couple of weeks were downers—with little, if any, positive feedback. So, after her initial web-research, she turned to her doctors and inundated them with page after page of questions. Why this procedure/medication/therapy and not that procedure/medication/therapy?

Michele's treatment plan included four rounds of neo-adjuvant (before surgery) chemotherapy from September through December 2001, followed by a radical mastectomy in January 2002 and then four more chemotherapy treatments with a different drug cocktail. In May she began radiation daily for 6 weeks.

A self-professed control freak, Michele had trouble sleeping throughout this period—she just couldn't be in the dark. Sleeping with the lights on helped, but she needed to fill up the space in her head, otherwise her mind reverted to "what ifs". With eyes too tired to read during the long nights, she discovered the next best thing—books on tape. During that ten-month period, she went through over 200 books, countless batteries, and more than once nearly asphyxiated herself by falling asleep with the headset cord wrapped around her neck. Borders Bookstore and the library were her preferred method of pain management therapy.

Chemo was the hardest part for Michele. After each treatment, she'd pace around her kitchen island, walking, walking, walking. *"It was so much more than just anxiety. Chemo is the closest to death you can be and still come back. I'd be pretty squirrelly for the first three days. Then on the fourth day after chemo, I would have to go to the Emergency Room for an IV drip to stop the nausea and vomiting. It would last 24 to 48 hours. This happened with all eight of my chemo treatments. Yet after the IV kicked in, we would stop at Dairy Queen on the way home for an ice cream cone. On the way to the hospital I'd be vomiting; on the way home I'd be eating ice cream! Go figure!"*

> ### *Note to Self:*
> *Some reminders hit you viscerally, others emotionally, still others spiritually. Cancer and its after-effects change the whole person, mind-body-spirit.*

A blue, Lysol-permeated scrub bucket was a constant companion in the backseat of Michele's car, just in case she felt nauseous. To this day, the smell of Lysol makes her instantly sick.

Michele's husband came to each and every doctor appointment and chemo treatment and kneeled beside her when the inevitable nausea followed. *"I'd be lying on the floor, embracing the toilet and my husband would promise me anything, anything I wanted, if I could just make it go away."*

Once the nausea subsided, Michele took him up on his promises and turned her Internet research skills to investigating cars. Prior to this, Michele had rarely even pumped her own gas, much less knew anything about cars, but she knew she wanted a convertible. When she finally found the car of her dreams, a black Chrysler Sebring convertible, she knew all about engines, tire sizes and gas mileage. The car dealer she contacted accepted her first low-ball offer when she told them she was a cancer patient and this was her reward for completing chemo.

In fact, the time spent researching kept her sane and her mind busy. Once the car was in the garage, she turned her attention to new appliances, including a dishwasher and flat cook-top stove since she loves to cook for family and friends. Even though the new "in" color for appliances was biscuit, Michele wanted a stove in almond to match her other appliances. After multiple dead ends, she finally sent an online plea directly to Frigidaire exclaiming, *"I've got breast cancer, can you help me?"* Miraculously, they unearthed an almond stove in a remote North Carolina warehouse and shipped it to a local retail store for delivery and installation.

"The drama queen in me was starting to take over, so I had to stop myself before my family did. I was using my cancer as a license to steal! I'd gotten a convertible, new appliances, a new laptop computer so I could work from home, a diamond anniversary band, a trip to Florida to visit family, and a trip to Arizona. JUST BECAUSE I WAS SICK!"

Note to Self:

Ask for what you need (translation: want) even if it seems outrageous at the time. Diversions can be an important element to healing.

Michele was prepared to lose her hair about 15 to 17 days after the start of chemo, but her bigger concern was that it coincided with homecoming weekend and her daughter was on court. Now homecoming weekend is a very big deal in every small town across the Midwest. Relieved and grateful she was on the fast track (her hair fell out only 13 days after chemo began), she first wore her wig in public to the football game. *"It was such a big day for my daughter, I didn't want anything to overshadow it for her.*

"And you know that family trip to Florida I mentioned earlier? When my daughter and I pulled up to my parents home in Florida, they all came out to meet us wearing, guess what? Wigs, of course. My Mom and Dad, my sister and her boyfriend, all wearing wigs…that was a sight!" Is it any wonder that Michele has such an I-will-get-through-this, in-love-with-life sense of humor?

"I'd had years of bad haircuts so losing my hair wasn't a big a deal for me. But when I asked my husband to help me shave the back of my head where I couldn't reach, he had tears in his eyes. Once finished, he pleaded, 'Never ask me to do that again.' It was the only thing he couldn't handle." Instead, Michele's daughter took over the grooming challenge, and became the make-up artist, teaching her mom how to draw on eyebrows once they, too, fell out.

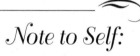

Note to Self:

We all have our limits. Sometimes we aren't even aware of them until we're right in the middle of a situation and realize it's outside our endurance capacity.

"On the day of my last chemo treatment, I was in the Oncology department, hooked up to an IV of the dreaded cocktail, while my baby sister was upstairs in the maternity ward giving birth. Now that's a miracle! I hoped and prayed that I could have a miracle, too."

I hoped and prayed that I could have a miracle, too.

Michele continued working in her HR position throughout her treatments. Her work gave her purpose and a focus for getting up and out. She thrived on chaos, particularly since the organization had been purchased by a new company about a month prior to her diagnosis. In hindsight, she realizes she became their *"designated poster child"*, an example of their compassionate, caring approach to employee relations, during an otherwise cynically-accepted transition. The new company continued her full salary and allowed Michele to work from home whenever necessary. She believes that the nature of the company, a healthcare provider, gave her co-workers more insight and compassion towards her illness.

Once her treatment and reconstruction surgery was complete, Michele decided to leave her full-time job. She now works as a temporary, part-time consultant to her former employer and has no interest in returning to the rat race. She guards her health and her time, selfishly picking and choosing her labors of love. She likes the flexibility to visit her daughter, now away at college, on the spur of the moment. She also loves to travel, and has recently adopted a dog named Molly, her new companion.

"One experience that I would not have wanted to live without, and cancer brought it to me, was walking the survivor lap at the local Relay For Life, sponsored by the American Cancer Society. My father was diagnosed last year with prostate cancer, so we both walked that survivor lap with tears in our eyes. We are already putting together our team for this year's event. It is truly a family affair."

We are already putting together our team for this year's event. It is truly a family affair.

Michele wonders if there will come a time when the cancer won't be front and center in her life and mind. Before finalizing vacation plans outside of the country, she was warned that a side effect of chemo is a compromised immune system, so she needed to be vigilant about the supply of clean drinking water. She's been warned to note any change in condition and to contact her doctor immediately if she experiences fevers, rashes or pain anywhere in her body (all signs of recurring inflammatory cancer). Is it any wonder Michele feels like she may be turning into a hypochondriac?

She is very clear that chemotherapy is not an option she will consider if her cancer recurs. Her decision is based on her own experience and the sense of personal injustice she felt. *"Chemotherapy stripped me of my self-respect. I would undergo radiation again, if possible, but I will not go through chemo again. I want my family to understand this."*

Cancer has changed Michele in many ways. She says she is kinder and more patient. To her own surprise, she has become more spiritual. One of the first people she called after her diagnosis was her parish priest, and during chemo, she found soothing comfort in her grandmother's rosary. That is, after she made a quick phone call to her friend, *"I know the one and ten thing, the Hail Mary's and the Our Father's, but I don't know the words for the beads in between."* Her friend's advice? *"I don't think it matters, just say what ever you want."* So Michele prays for time. Not so much for herself, but for her husband (who she is certain will turn into a hermit without her) and for her daughter, who needs her mom around for as long as possible.

As I prepare to e-mail Michele my version of her story, I give her a quick call to catch up on things. She's just returned from a family vacation in the Caribbean, took her daughter back to college yesterday and she's taking her dad (who's just recovered from a diabetic coma two weeks ago and is already feeling perky) to a casino tomorrow. She wonders if I can give her a couple of days to react and respond. This is one busy woman! I mention that my one-year anniversary mammogram is next week, and she notes that she has just had her annual full-body CT scans today. Michele is supposed to hear back on Friday but told her family and friends it will be next week before she gets results. *"I need personal time to process and absorb whatever the results might be."* We hold our breaths in unison and wait for answers to come.

Reshaping

My most vivid childhood memories always include a kaleidoscope. Entering my grandmother's woodstove-warmed parlor, I'd race to pick up the treasured cardboard tube first. I would spend most of my visit peering into the tiny peephole, fascinated by the changing colors and patterns.

For my 50th birthday, my husband gifted me with an exquisite stained glass kaleidoscope filled with a rainbow of gem-colored glass pieces. Daily, I'd lift it from its stand and gaze deeply into its recesses, wanting to capture forever the jeweled, geometrically-perfect formations. Unknown to either of us at that point, cancer was growing in my left breast.

Cancer is often called a life-shattering illness. The better terminology is life reshaping. Just as our bodies may take a new form (whether through scarring or through silicone), our lives are changed forever. With time, our initial physical and emotional brokeness is replaced with a richer, deeper, brighter, clearer perspective. We know life's fragility and pick up the bits and pieces to recast a new life mold. We know that faith, family and friends are life's most precious jewels. Our priorities shifted, they become a brilliant configuration at the center of our lives.

Kaleidoscope

bits and pieces
form and reform

crystals and gems
no two patterns alike

Ah, a beautiful one!

gone in a glance
powerless to bring it back

no one else will ever see
what I've seen

one slight shift and
it's gone

—Christy L. Schwan

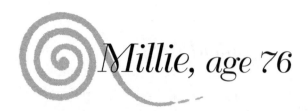

Millie, age 76

*U*nassuming, quiet and soft-spoken, Millie always has a ready smile. Her favorite colors are peach and mauve, the colors of sunrise, and she enjoys reading, gardening and knitting. Her patience, stoicism and optimism are quickly revealed as she succinctly describes her life, *"My husband died two years ago. After he had a massive stroke in 1994, I was his caregiver for seven years. Even though he was aphasic, he kept his sense of humor and was ambulatory until the end, so he never was a burden. He was a widower with two boys when we married, and we had two girls and three more boys of our own. I worked in various secretarial positions until 1994, except for the 17 years after I married and raised a family."*

Millie was 76 in late summer 2001 when her cancer was first diagnosed. One morning while making the bed, she tripped and ended up in the hospital with a broken hip. While confined, Millie's doctor providentially ordered a variety of other tests, including a mammogram. She'd always been healthy and of strong German stock, so the only other surgery she'd ever had was a tonsillectomy as a child. Because she's also a procrastinator, this was her very first mammogram. It revealed a tumor approximately 1$^1/_2$ centimeters in diameter.

Cancer cells were discovered and she elected to have a lumpectomy. Millie was adamantly against a mastectomy the first time around. She felt she was just too healthy to need it at this stage. Like many women, there was little history of breast cancer in her family. Her aunt, who's now in her

*N*ote to Self:

The diagnosis can quickly undermine your self-image of health, initially taking away your self-confidence.

The Blue Tattoo Club

mid-80s, had been diagnosed about 25 years prior, but there were no other occurrences.

Millie had no choice but to bring her husband along with her to every appointment, every test, every procedure. Since Tom couldn't express himself at that point, Millie was never able to find out exactly what he thought about all that activity. She mentions that the only time anyone could understand him was when he got mad and then he'd let out a well-articulated *"damn"*, reminding them all that he still had an opinion.

The lumpectomy revealed that the cancer had already spread to her lymph nodes. Before deciding on the next step, she took nearly three months to research her options. Her doctor was very careful to explain the alternatives. Millie asked lots of questions and talked with many other women. *"I was most afraid of telling my family that I had cancer. Once I did that and decided on a treatment, I pretty much accepted it. The low point was after additional cancer was found and I had to decide what should be done. My family and my faith have been my support."*

She was particularly interested in reconstructive surgery and ultimately made the decision to have a mastectomy with immediate breast replacement surgery. Millie just smiles when she says, *"It was ego. I wanted to look good and I just asked myself 'why not?'."*

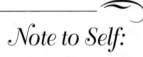

Note to Self:

"Why not?" is as good an answer as any. Try it on for size sometime.

She decided to have a saline prosthesis at the time of the mastectomy, but her medical oncologist never liked the shape of it. After a year it started to leak and in November 2002, it was removed and another one inserted. *"My oncologist commented that I had one very perky breast and one not so perky. They haven't perfected making an aging and sagging one to match my surviving one!"*

Millie chose to forego chemo and radiation, but did have 8 weeks of physical therapy following her mastectomy. *"The walking wall was helpful in regaining my range of motion even though it was intense."* Neither Millie, nor her family, ever relied much on medication although she does take Vitamin E and is on Tamoxifin. As a former yoga student, Millie did participate in transcendental meditation as part of a study conducted by St. Joseph's Hospital in Chicago. Finding it both relaxing and a stress-reliever, she still practices it occasionally on her own. It taught her to take everything one day at a time and not to sweat the small stuff.

Millie's seven children provided most of her support and helped relieve her from some of her caregiving responsibilities while she was recovering herself. She was taken by surprise at the number of friends and acquaintances who expressed their concern and compassion for her. *"I hug people a lot more now, in spite of my German upbringing, and I don't confuse support with sympathy. I did grieve in the beginning and felt very sorry for myself. But I made up my mind to get going because I was too busy to be self-concerned. I don't know if it is because of my stoicism, but I never felt that my cancer was life threatening, especially after deciding to have the mastectomy."*

Millie pressed a smooth stone into my hand after church services one morning. *"This is for you from my breast cancer support group; we're thinking about you."* Not until later that day do I notice the word HOPE engraved on its surface. It sits in a zen sand garden on my office desk, a gentle daily reminder.

"I had 47 years of marriage to a special person and am now just enjoying the remainder of life. I've always wanted to travel. So to celebrate my recovery, I will fulfill this dream in August when a son and a daughter and I will go to Australia to visit another son who lives there and is married with two children."

Transformation

Rather than chisel away at granite blocks, some sculptors use plaster molds to create the images they envision. I compare this to the compressed foam mold that the technicians formed around me as part of the preparation for radiation treatment. Fitting like a glove, the mold was designed to hold my body immobile while the radiation precisely hit its potentially cancerous target.

Nestling into the initially awkward position became second nature. Those few minutes of quiet aloneness, with the technicians safely behind protective barriers, were womb-like. Despite the buzz of the machines, it was a time for repose and reflection. My mind floated over the life events leading up to that point and I'd mentally mark another day off my therapy calendar. Since my appointments were the last scheduled, I'd typically be out by 4:30 p.m. (hours before my pre-cancerous workaholic daily timetable). I'd drive home unhurriedly, anticipating the comfort of my husband's arms and the family room couch.

This mold was uniquely me, only mine, always waiting when I walked into the room. It was my personal cocoon, transforming me into a cancer-free, light-as-air creature. That's certainly how I felt on my last day of treatment. I'd accomplished a goal I'd never set out to achieve, the passage from invincibility to vulnerability to courage to strength.

The end result? A well-lived woman, having cast aside her mold, who now approaches the delicacy of life with the solidity, fortitude and grace of a Venus de Milo.

—*Christy L. Schwan*

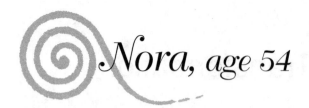

Nora, age 54

*N*ora is loving, kind and compassionate—a reader, gardener, music lover and bookkeeper. An expressive, self-confessed Type A personality, she was a workaholic until faced with breast cancer. She loves a neat, clean house, hanging sheets outside to dry and then putting the air-freshened linens right back on the beds. Unable to have children of their own, her husband's daughter has become hers as well. Their young grandson is the joy of their lives and melts their hearts each time they hear his voice.

Due to a family history of breast cancer, Nora had routine mammograms for twenty years. In October 2001, she was scheduled for rotator cuff surgery and decided to have her annual mammogram first, since she wouldn't be able to assume the positions for quite a while after her shoulder surgery. The mammograms and ultrasounds were followed by a stereotactic core biopsy the next day. Her cancer was labeled as Stage 1, but the doctor still felt that treatment needed to begin quickly because the type of cancer could be aggressive. He recommended a lumpectomy followed by chemotherapy and radiation.

After a massive lumpectomy, the pathology reports confirmed that her cancer was Estrogen-Receptor-Positive and very aggressive. A second surgery to remove lymph nodes was done two weeks later with great news—all 26 lymph nodes were clear!

Chemotherapy began two weeks after that and continued every three weeks for five months. The sheer exhaustion was as difficult for Nora as was the nausea, vomiting, diarrhea, and constipation. *"A couple of times, I didn't take my anti-nausea medication as promptly as I should have and I dearly paid a price for it. I would get extremely nauseated just coming into the parking lot of the hospital, much less having to come in for labs, etc. I didn't know if I'd be physically strong enough to see it all through. I felt like I had lost much of the control of my life so my surgeon asked me to take just one day at a time, and get through that, and then tomorrow do it all over again."*

The evening before each chemotherapy, Nora lined up all of the meds she needed for the next several days on the kitchen counter along with a notepad to record what and when she took each item. It usually consisted of two kinds of anti-nausea pills, stool softeners, and Milk of Magnesia (Vanilla Crème and Cherry were her flavors of choice). After about ten days, she'd put the supply away until the next session.

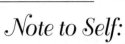

Note to Self:

Milk of Magnesia and Gatorade take on a whole new meaning once you've been through chemotherapy. Once chemo is over, don't hesitate to banish them from your medicine cabinet or pantry forever.

Then each morning before she left for chemo, she would dust and vacuum the bedroom and put fresh linens on the bed so that when she came home from the hospital she could climb immediately into a nice, soothing cocoon. Since she was so exhausted during chemo, Nora spent a lot of time in bed and this ritual became very important to her. Even though her husband offered to help, most of the time she preferred to do it herself. It helped take her mind off her upcoming treatment and gave her something constructive to do.

During chemo, Nora was encouraged (no, actually told) to drink a large quantity of liquids each day to stay hydrated and to flush the chemicals through her body. She'd always liked water, but it became extremely difficult to get down when she was so nauseated, so her oncologist suggested Gatorade as an alternative. Gatorade seemed even worse so the doctor suggested diluting it with 7-up, ginger ale, water, etc. Her husband bought every new flavor and tried a variety of methods to make it appealing but no matter what flavor, what pretty color or temperature it was, she just couldn't down it. Her doctor even suggested putting it in a shot glass and just taking a few sips whenever she walked through the kitchen. It began to seem like every time her husband came near her, he had something for her to drink.

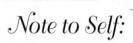

Note to Self:

Kind of reminds you of the first time you got drunk; the very thought of that specific drink can still make you gag years later.

"My husband, Rick, kept me going during the hard times. He would help me shower even though I didn't want to bother and then after a few days into my chemo, he'd make me go for a ride with him just to get out of the house. We'd often end up doing lunch somewhere and I'd make an attempt to eat as best I could. It was easy to just push the food around my plate in my own home, but the starving-Chinese-children image was ingrained in my brain, so I felt obligated to try to eat everything. He'd let me stay in bed much of the time, but on nice days, he'd coax me out on the patio to keep him company. When my nieces, daughter or other special people called, he'd give me the phone even though I didn't think I was up to talking with anyone. He made me laugh and hugged me when it became a tear. Some days I followed him from room to room when I didn't really want to be alone, but he never seemed to mind. He always had a ready smile and blanket to cover me when I got chilled and then helped my get it off quickly when the hot flashes came!"

Once the chemo was over, seven weeks of radiation therapy were scheduled, but another mammogram was required first. More mammograms, ultrasounds and another stereotactic core biopsy finally revealed, to her shock and disbelief, that cancer had recurred. Although the diagnosing physician recommended another lumpectomy, her surgeon recommended a complete mastectomy immediately. Nora had already come to that conclusion; she couldn't live from month to month in dread of another recurrence. So in May 2002, she had a complete mastectomy.

"The surgeon who did my lumpectomy, axillary node dissection and my mastectomy has been truly compassionate, as has been his staff. He allows me to shed tears when I need to and gives me a gentle hug to let me know he cares. He continues to give me hope without being patronizing and allows me to discuss my true feelings regarding my present and future treatment options. When I was in the hospital for the reconstruction surgeries and subsequent complications, he stopped by the operating holding room just to say hello, hold my hand and wish me well. I finally had the rotator cuff surgery after 2 years and while the anesthesiologist was preparing a nerve block, he held my hand and talked with me until it was done. He then went out and talked with my husband for a while—and he wasn't even doing my surgery."

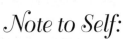

Note to Self:

Don't be rushed into treatment with doctors with whom you're not comfortable. Ask for referrals from others and keep asking questions until you get answers that you understand. Choose a doctor who will be honest, forthright, realistic, yet compassionate--they do exist. Trust your doctors, but if you don't agree with their recommendations, discuss it with them.

Nora's lowest point was while she was waiting for the biopsy to confirm whether the cancer had recurred or not. Because it was over a weekend, she had to wait for the results for several days. Still in shock that more cancer was suspected, it was extremely difficult for her when it recurred. *"It's not that I thought I would never get breast cancer, especially with a family history of it. It's just so hard to believe that it is all really happening and never seems to end. I didn't allow myself to grieve for the first several months—I was just too busy trying to keep everything normal. I grieved when cancer recurred. Although my family let me shed many, many tears, they kept me focused on getting through this. I truly never felt that I was mutilated or no longer a real woman. Losing a breast was more just a daily reminder that I had cancer—something I can't get away from or forget about."* Her oncologist prescribed a low dose, anti-depressant which made a significant difference and allowed her to gain emotional control to get through some of the roughest days.

It's not that I thought I would never get breast cancer, especially with a family history of it. It's just so hard to believe that it is all really happening and never seems to end.

Prior to the mastectomy, Nora met with a plastic surgeon to discuss reconstruction options. During the mastectomy surgery, he implanted a tissue expander in her chest to begin the reconstruction. She opted to have a saline implant put in—she wanted to be able to get dressed the same way each day that she had for the past 45 years and didn't want to have to deal with a breast prosthesis. For the next several months, she went to the doctor's office weekly for saline injections into the tissue expander.

Unfortunately, her body reacted by forming excessive scar tissue. She had to have another surgery to try to remove the scar tissue so that her skin would stretch more easily. During this time, she was also undergoing another four months of chemotherapy. Finally, in November 2002, a saline implant was placed in her chest and although it isn't quite as large as her natural breast, she's very pleased with the results. Due to the scar tissue problems, she will probably not have the breast finished--the nipple and areola--which is disappointing. But she trusts the judgment of her surgeon and is confident that he has her best interests in mind. In December 2002, Nora began the Tamoxifen regime and the hot flashes resumed. (She'd been on HRT for twelve years prior to her breast surgery due to a need for a hysterectomy at 45.)

After her mastectomy, Nora and her husband took a getaway trip to the lake area of northern Wisconsin before her second round of chemotherapy was to begin. Once her chemo treatments ended, they flew to Texas to see their young grandson. Even though she was exhausted, the trip was just what she needed-- a two-year-old grandson can make it all better.

Nora's employer granted her medical leaves as she needed them, so she took two weeks off after each chemo treatment. Going back to work until the next treatment brought some normalcy to her life. *"I enjoy working and being around others, so this was a great help to me. The time off was unpaid with no benefits, but I was never pressured to come in when I wasn't up to it. I've since been told that everyone was so impressed with the class and dignity with which I handled myself and left my problems at home. I do feel good about that, although there were some days when I really could have used a hug."*

Nora regrets not allowing her friends to help. Many called initially and urged her to call if she needed anything, but Nora never asked. Often she felt so sick that she didn't feel like talking with anyone at all— she was just trying to keep going as best she could. She's now hurt that many of their close friends have not stayed in touch and others have told her that it was hitting too close to home, so they just couldn't handle it.

Note to Self:

Be careful what you don't ask for. Others may wait for you to take the lead, to show them what to do. They can be torn between wanting to help and not wanting to interfere. Let your family and friends help when they offer.

"One morning when I had just started losing a lot of my hair, a dear friend from Florida called and all I could do was cry. I told her that she didn't call long-distance just to hear me cry and she said if it helped, she'd listen to me cry as long as I wanted to. She doesn't judge me when I'm having a bad day and lets me know it's okay. I found that most of my other friends only wanted me to be laughing and joking around like normal. If I got serious or quiet, they were uncomfortable.

"You have to keep up a good attitude." "At least you're alive." "There are people a lot worse off than you." "One good thing about having breast cancer is that you got curly hair out of it." "You'll look back on

this and be glad it happened." Nora considered keeping a Top 20 List of Stupid Things People Have Said, but chose to let their comments slide off.

Nora's sister-in-law, a breast cancer survivor, came down from Minnesota several times just to be with Nora for a day or so. The day of the mastectomy, she surprised Nora when she came out of the recovery room. After a big hug, she made a few meals to have on hand and then left the next morning for another six-hour drive home. Nora's daughter came up from Texas several times and just took over—sometimes rearranging things so that they'd have to laughingly call her just to find out where she'd put them! Knowing Nora's favorite treat, she'd hang the bed sheets outside to dry. That's one smell Nora couldn't get enough of. Her nieces offered to come down but she usually told them no, because she worried about them driving alone for six hours at night. *"I realize now that I deprived them of a chance to help me when they really wanted to."*

Nora has had a difficult time with a severe case of *"chemo brain"* caused by all of the chemotherapy and the multiple surgeries. Her doctors tell her to just give it time, that it is reversible but she struggles with short-term memory loss and tends to interchange words incorrectly. She's not patient with herself, so her doctors have recommended that she de-stress her life as much as possible to minimize frustration. Laughing is one way that Nora keeps her stress levels low.

"A friend was going through breast cancer a few months after I had recurred. We made fun of our hair (or lack thereof), the stupid remarks people made to us, etc. I drove her to some of her radiation treatments and one day in the car, she said 'Stop me if I've told you this already. You know with my chemo brain, I can't remember what

I've said.' I replied, 'With my chemo brain, I wouldn't know the difference anyway.' We then assumed that we probably had the SAME CONVERSATION each time we rode together, but who cares? We walked into the Oncology department laughing our heads off. I guess we needed that.

"Another episode was when I had an appointment with my oncologist for a three month checkup. He's a tremendously caring man, but always runs late. I had to run to the restroom several

> ## *Note to Self:*
> Call a friend and ask them to wash and line dry your sheets—a simple, inexpensive indulgence? Yes! Think about it. You can't help but breathe deeply and fully when you bring them inside, whip them in the air and wrap them around the mattress. Cocoon yourself inside for a whole body experience.

times out of nervousness. It was a good examination and the results were finally positive so we decided to go to Smith Brothers for a celebration dinner. Once again, I used the restroom at the restaurant.

"After arriving home, I decided to get into something more comfortable. I have to wear a partial prosthesis due to the problems I've had with my implant. As I was going to put the prosthesis back into its box, I realized that it wasn't in my bra. Somehow, it had fallen out. I quickly checked my voicemail, assuming that I must have lost it at the hospital and they would have called to tell me that they had it. No voice mail! I began to panic that somehow I had lost it at Smith Brothers—maybe in the restroom or maybe even as I was walking out of the restaurant. What should I do? My husband said to call the restaurant and ask if anyone had found something "odd". Can you just imagine what their reaction might have been?

"The prosthesis is quite expensive and I was trying to quickly calculate how many lunches I might have to forego to save for a replacement. I finally realized that I really did have to make the call (or at least try to get my husband to do it). How would I phrase it?

Then, my husband asked me if I had already put it in its box and just didn't remember because of "chemo brain". I thought he was just trying to buy me some time, so I looked. Would you believe it was resting comfortably in the box? I don't know if I even bothered to put it into my bra before I left for the appointment, but at least I didn't have to make any calls!"

After each surgery, Nora wasn't able to shower for a few days due to all of the dressings and sutures, etc. Her husband either realized how much better she'd feel after a shower, felt sorry for her, or knew that SHE REALLY NEEDED A SHOWER. A retired Industrial Tech instructor, he came up with the idea

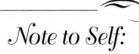

Note to Self:

Nora is allergic to adhesive tape but didn't have any problems with duct tape. Is there an idea here for use in the medical field?

of taping plastic grocery bags to her chest so that she could let the water run over her entire body with little risk of getting her dressings wet. After trial and error, they found that good old silver duct tape seemed to hold better than other adhesives when it got wet. It wasn't pretty, but it was functional!

The number of bags necessary for each shower was based on the "quality" of each bag and if she had drains to enclose as well. Sometimes they got a little fancier when she really needed a longer shower for her mental well-being. She'd then insert her arm through the handles of the bag, assuring it a little more durability. Her husband then taped all of the edges to her chest and underarm area. It took a few minutes to get all of this in place before showering and then more time once she got out. Then they'd peel off the bags and tape while still in the shower to avoid getting the floor and mats totally wet. Due to the significant usage of grocery bags, they needed to shop more often and keep the bags lighter so that they wouldn't tear or get too distorted. This might be a clue to why Nora gained weight after her surgeries!

The Blue Tattoo Club

"Tubing was placed into my chest during surgery to allow body fluids to drain while I was recovering. It was uncomfortable under my arm and it would get pinched off or pulled if I moved wrong or when I was trying to sleep. The bulb had to be lower than the tubing so that gravity could allow the fluid to flow properly, so it had to be pinned to my clothing. More than once, I pinned the bulb to my slacks and then "forgot" when I had to use the bathroom and pulled my slacks down before remembering to unpin the bulb first. It only takes a few times of doing that before your memory gets sharper! When I first had the dressings, Rick helped me pin it on, drain the tubes and measure the contents as it was awkward for me to handle and I was still quite sore. My drains were in longer than normal—a few weeks at least— and the area around the tube became irritated. It sure felt good to have them removed.

"My life gifts are the awareness of unconditional love and support from my family for so many years and especially during my struggle with breast cancer. What a wonderful gift it is to know that others are praying for us through our tough times. Another gift is realizing that I've had a wonderful life and although I'm not certain that I will be a breast cancer survivor, I am comfortable that the time I've had on this earth has been a blessing.

> ## Note to Self:
> Be kind to yourself and allow the emotions to come. You have the right to be angry, sad, or depressed about what's happening to you. Listen to what your body needs and follow its lead.

"I must honestly admit that, at first, I did not have many fears. I felt that the cancer was caught early and that recovery/survival will be the end result. My recurrence has made me wary of that now. My greatest fear is that I will not live long enough to see my grandson grow up, or my nieces' families grow."

Nora's physical therapist deals predominantly in breast cancer rehabilitation. She's been good for Nora's spirit as well as her body, validating many of her concerns about treatments, ongoing side effects and the possibility of not surviving breast cancer. Nora has spent time getting her affairs in order in case the cancer recurs. Her therapist recognizes that Nora's need to talk about death doesn't mean that she's wishing for it.

In February 2003, during a follow-up visit for her implant, Nora's surgeon found a mass under her arm and recommended biopsy and surgery to remove it. Her oncologist agreed but thought that as long as the mass had to come out anyway, it made more sense to biopsy it afterwards instead of going through two surgeries. At the same time, Nora's husband was in the hospital undergoing extensive heart surgery with complications, so they decided to wait until he'd recovered. In April 2003, she had another surgery to remove the mass. Thankfully, it was not malignant and had not entered her lymph system.

Note to Self:

It's hard to be upbeat for another person when you're experiencing breast cancer. Cut yourself some slack, give yourself a break, save guilt for another time and place.

"My husband is truly my soulmate, even after almost 30 years, and through each adversity in our lives has continually assured me that he will always be there for me. Throughout my ongoing struggle with breast cancer, he has not wavered in his loving care and support. He is my rock and if it weren't for him, I don't know if I'd have come through this journey as well. He has gone to every doctor/lab/chemotherapy appointment and has been continually upbeat on my prognosis—even after my recurrence—but has also been honest, realistic, and comforting. He has shared many of my tears and is gentle enough to just let them come and hold me when I need it. He has had major health problems during this same period

but continues to keep me going. At times, I feel guilty that I have not been as upbeat for him as I should have been."

In July 2003, after a couple of months of knee pain, Nora was diagnosed with vascular degeneration of the knee, possibly caused by her extensive chemotherapy. An MRI revealed that the cancer had not gone to her knee, but she did need to spend about eight weeks on crutches. Slowly the leg has improved and she's hopeful that it will continue to do so.

"I've learned that I am much stronger and more resilient than I ever thought I could be. I was able to keep it all together especially when I was among others, no matter how terrible I actually felt. I only let down with my family and special friends. I also learned how much faith I truly have. I've never gotten angry and asked 'Why me?' I realize how blessed my life has been. I also learned to be more content and not feel that I have to always being doing something. My priorities have changed a great deal—my family has always come first, but now they mean even more to me."

I've learned that I am much stronger and more resilient than I ever thought I could be. I was able to keep it all together especially when I was among others, no matter how terrible I actually felt.

Nora takes life more seriously now, even though her family can still set her off into giggling spasms. She's become more aware of others who are hurting and appreciates those who have cared for her. Even though she's been disappointed by the lack of concern from some friends and feels like it's hardened her, in her heart she knows that she would still help out if something happened to them. That's the real Nora—the Nora that will never change.

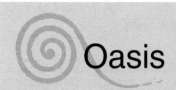# Oasis

"Find Your Own Oasis". Just a line from a magazine advertisement. I read it once and an image flashes through my mind. I go back and read it again. I get a pen and write down the phrase. Dust, grit and sand are all elements in the picture. Without that point of reference, there is little need for a refuge. If the surrounding terrain was lush and verdant, there wouldn't be a noticeable difference or need for a haven. We'd walk right past it.

So why did that phrase strike me? The ad intimated that the oasis could be found at their exclusive spa. I suspect that we each harbor our own internal oasis. That place we go to wash away the residue of regret, refresh ourselves and drink in the waters of renewal.

I sometimes find my oasis when I read. Sometimes when I write. Sometimes when I inspect my flower garden for signs of new growth. Sometimes when I soak in the tub. Sometimes when I veg on the couch. Sometimes when I talk with a friend. Sometimes when I talk with God. Sometimes when I talk with my dog. God forbid, there have even been a few isolated incidents when I've found it in the middle of washing the dishes.

I wrote the above paragraphs years before my breast cancer diagnosis, at a time when my definition of an oasis meant a retreat from the unyielding demands of building a business and raising a family. Then breast cancer crept in and created an instant desert in my life. Like sand, the sadness permeated every crevice of my being. It dried me out. My tears turned to dust and then I had no tears left to cry.

But yet when I was finally able to look up and in, my internal oasis hadn't evaporated: it had become wider and more vivid. The littlest things in my life became and remain the most refreshing, most revitalizing parts in my life. But now I would add: my husband's arms, my mother's hug, my father's prayers, my daughter's laugh, my son's voice, my granddaughter's smile.

—Christy L. Schwan

The Blue Tattoo Club

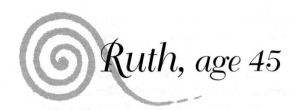

Ruth, age 45

Ruth is an animated, energetic, talkative, open, compassionate, yet no-nonsense, caregiver in her role as a Lutheran Associate in Ministry. She has a close relationship with her two adult daughters who think of her as a warrior. She met her husband, Jim, on a blind date and he still likes to brag that he told his friend the next day, *"I just met the girl I'm going to marry!"* He teases her gently about her lingering memory loss and occasionally calls her a dumb blonde to which she responds serenely, *"Yeah, but I try not to be."* She considers herself a strong woman, yet when she's in a doctor's office, she often can't stop crying.

Ruth was in her mid-40s when she found the lump right before her scheduled biennial mammogram seven years ago. Like so many other women, she had no family history of breast cancer. Her physicians believe that the growth of the large tumor was accelerated by the estrogen replacement drugs she was taking for premature menopause, osteoporosis and a heart condition that runs in her family.

Note to Self:

How do you get past feeling like you should have known? Especially if there is no family history of breast cancer? The myth of the all-knowing, all-seeing, all-feeling female is just that —a myth.

The diagnosis was announced by a phone call from her physician in early February. She underwent two biopsies where the doctors removed a 5$\frac{1}{2}$ centimeter invasive lump. Her surgeries were performed before sentinel node biopsies were common practice. Six nodes were removed and came back negative, yet there was uncertainty about whether enough nodes had been tested, particularly since in situ cells had been found at the margins.

Once surgery was completed, Ruth was considered for a research test group but ultimately chose not to participate. It would have changed the timing of her treatments, interfering with her scheduled worship services. Her next decision point was to choose which chemotherapy route to take—a decision which did not come easily. The tumor size led her to take a more aggressive action than her oncologist thought necessary. *"I decided to go the whole nine yards up front, at the same time wondering whether I was making a martyr of myself. But I did not want to live with any regrets."*

Early in our conversation, Ruth mentions the blanket of guilt that she carries with her, having grown up in a household where mistakes were viewed as sins. As if reminding herself, she tells me that nothing would have changed even if they'd found the tumor earlier. Had the cancer progressed to her lymph nodes, the blanket would have been thicker and heavier.

On April 1st, Ruth began chemotherapy with an almost toxic level of Adriamycin repeated every three weeks. Since Sunday is her big workday, each session started on Monday morning with an anti-nausea and relaxation prescription. The doctors did not want Ruth throwing up, but she was incapable of even keeping water down during the treatments. Ultimately, fluids had to be administered intravenously in a darkened, private room, so that Ruth could be sedated enough to sleep through the entire process. This process lasted a full day on Monday and half days on Tuesdays and Wednesdays. By Saturday night, Ruth was able to participate in evening worship services. *"I'm proud to say I never missed a Saturday or Sunday service! Since our pastor was on sabbatical at that time, I felt my presence was important for our members."*

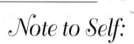

Note to Self:

Studies have shown that women who experienced severe morning sickness while pregnant are also more prone to nausea with chemo.

Halfway through Ruth's chemo regimen, her younger daughter was finishing her senior year of high school. *"There are some life events you do not want to interfere with, no matter what your health condition is. I did not want the memory of my daughter's high school graduation burdened with my cancer-related side effects. This was her day, so I delayed one of my chemo treatments for a week, in spite of my anxiety."*

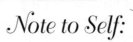

Note to Self:

Life goes on during chemo— yours and everyone else's. Sometimes you can avoid the disruption of life events, sometimes not.

Ruth has always been *"into hair"*. It was very hard when hers began falling out while attending Parents' Weekend at her daughter's college. *"I'd brought my wig along—I had a sense that it would happen that weekend. Once it started, it just kept coming, and coming, and coming… My girls were 18 and 21 at the time, so they could relate to my loss. I'll always remember the three-way hug and their tender affirmations of love in that tiny hotel bathroom.*

"Believe it or not, I looked really good during chemo. I had a lovely bald head with no bumps (although no one but my family ever saw it), my complexion was clear and rosy, and I lost the extra weight I'd been trying to lose for years. Although shopping for a wig was hard, I had to do it since I do NOT look good in hats. We must have done a good job picking out a believable hair replacement, since some people never knew I ever wore a wig. We did take pictures of my bald head, which I now share with other cancer patients.

"I also wrote a letter to our insurance company appealing their denial of payment for my wig. It didn't change their decision, but that wig was as important to my overall health and wellness as a breast prosthesis is to other women. It's much easier to disguise a breast than it is baldness."

Ruth has learned a lot about breast cancer over these seven years and noted that certain breast cancers feed on estrogen. In some ways, those tumors are better than others because medical professionals have more ways to battle them. On the other hand, doctors are concerned about even small doses of estrogen for women with these types of cancers. It's a hard consequence. Ruth had been on estrogen replacement medication for about 18 months and had to stop cold-turkey, immediately interrupting her sleep patterns, her memory and her emotional balance. *"The multiple layers of change have a lingering impact on your physical, emotional and sexual well-being. As testosterone levels drop in tandem, many women experience extreme vaginal dryness and a loss of sex-drive, leaving them feeling non-sexual, even asexual. It's not about love. You just don't think about sex anymore."*

With her bodily estrogen wiped out nearly overnight, chemo brain was exacerbated. She wasn't able to focus enough to read an article or watch TV, much less read a book. She's an avid Elvis fan, so her husband bought her vintage videos, but she couldn't even watch those. When she discussed her concerns with her doctor, his response was indifferent, *"Well, what do you want me to do about it?"*

Ruth had always given 120% at work but decided to use her limited energy to deal with people rather than with paper. Sermon preparation was a particular challenge—requiring a level of concentration she just didn't have. She gave herself permission not to function at even 100% and quickly realized that even 85% was okay.

After each chemo treatment, Ruth's serotonin levels dropped, causing depression, anxiety and irrational fears to the point of debilitation. For the first time in her life, she could not talk or motivate herself out of the depression and grew concerned that she'd never be able to fully function again. *"I believe the disease and the subsequent treatment create a physical reaction in your brain that destabilizes your emotional equilibrium. Cancer has invaded your body and you have a different sense of impending disaster and vulnerability than ever before."* With medication, treatment, counseling and time, Ruth has regained much of her former self. Even though her family is hesitant, she still takes anti-depressants for anxiety attacks. *"It has been difficult for them to grasp that this is*

> ## Note to Self:
> *Every person handles things differently. Don't compare yourself or allow others to compare you to other breast cancer patients.*

not about pessimism versus optimism. They're now beginning to acknowledge that it is a physical not an emotional condition."

While moving her daughter back home to Wisconsin from Pensacola, Ruth noticed a billboard advertising Graceland—an impetuous, wildly invigorating detour resulted. *"We went on all the tours and we thought we'd whip right through the car museum but instead we read every line. We even bought the cheesy picture of the two of us standing at the gate. I was just so glad to be alive. I've learned the importance of playtime with my daughters."*

Having completed the prescribed five years on Tamoxifin, Ruth is no longer taking cancer prevention drugs. That was a hard step for her to take even though her doctor determined additional drugs were not necessary. *"While I was on Tamoxifin, I felt like I was still battling cancer. Now that the treatment plan is completed, it is mentally hard for me to take no action. I ask myself, 'Now what?'. I do continue to be involved with my support group. I think it's important for women to be able to name their demons and to have permission to say, 'This stinks!'. My role in our support group is to balance the voice of optimism with the voice of realism."*

The greatest blessing that Ruth experienced is God's help throughout her treatment. She realizes that she's devoted too much of her time to work. *"It is possible for someone else to do my job, but no one else can be my husband's wife or my daughters' mother."*

Rituals are habits that develop a deeper meaning over time. Ruth hadn't realized she'd developed a comforting, healing ritual until we delved further into her story over dinner one night. An avid frog collector for over 20 years, she noticed a cute little wooly frog in the hospital gift shop window as they were wheeling her out after her surgery. Her husband gladly bought it for her, even though it felt more like a teddy bear than a frog. *"He had a pink cord around his neck and was the cutest, cuddliest, happiest little frog I'd ever seen (and I have literally hundreds of frogs.) I named him Ponder. Due to the post-surgical drains, I had to lie on one side and keep my arm down when I was in bed. I tucked Ponder under my surgery arm as a support cushion. I continued to snuggle with Ponder throughout my treatments and for a long time afterward. He still sits in our bedroom, all matted and rumpled, as a symbol of my husband's constant love and support."*

What are Ruth's life lessons? She's let go of thinking that looks are what counts—she's learned to love her wrinkles. She's happy with maintaining a heart-healthy weight even if it's not reflected in a single-digit-dress-size. She carries less guilt and complains less about the little things. She's stopped crucifying herself, giving herself permission to feel good and bad. When she's having a bad hair day, she reminds herself that at least she has hair. Her family helps her celebrate by raising money for Relay for Life, knowing that their research keeps women alive much longer. She finds joy in each new day and she religiously signs all of her cards—"CELEBRATE LIFE!"

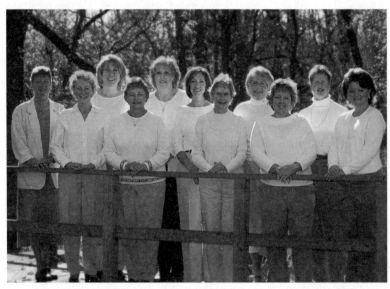

(Left to Right) Lynn, Christy, Janet, Gloria, Jennifer, Karen, Millie, Ruth, Michele, Nora, Connie

The Blue Tattoo Club

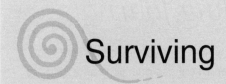

Surviving

Every day is a gift. Each breath is a blessing.

No matter how long I live after the diagnosis, I am a breast cancer survivor. It makes no difference whether my personal metaphor is that of a battling warrior/hero, a serene, long-suffering saint, or a reluctant just-let-me-get-through-this participant. If I survive with my spirit unbroken, if my essence is essentially intact, then I am whole. Wholeness is less about body parts than it is about spirit.

I hope you've had a glimpse into the spirits of the women profiled here. Severely tested but never crushed, our spirits were enriched as we tapped into wellsprings of strength we didn't know we had. Breast cancer guided us to become more grateful, more introspective, more focused, more trusting, more spiritual. These gifts have shaped us tangibly and will lead us down paths that we might not have taken before. We are connected forever as members of the Blue Tattoo Club.

We leave you with the words to the song "How Could Anyone" by Libby Roderick (on the recording "If You See a Dream" by Libby Roderick or "Songs for the Inner Child" by Shaina Noll):

How could anyone ever tell you
you were anything less than beautiful?
How could anyone ever tell you you were less than whole?
How could anyone fail to notice that your loving is a miracle?
How deeply you're connected to my soul?

—Christy L. Schwan

Healing Journal

You may find it healing to write about your own personal experience with breast cancer. Use these questions as a guide to help you explore your own reactions, thoughts and concerns.

1 _____ is my favorite color because...

2 I am...

3 I take care of myself by...

4 I let other people show they care about me by letting them...

5 I let my emotions out by...

6 I should live because...

7 I'm angry because...

8 I am afraid that...

9 During the hard times, it helps if...

10 The lowest point for me was...

11 The most meaningful thing that someone said to me was...

12 The stupidest thing that someone said to me was...

13 The funniest thing that happened to me was...

14 A ritual or habit that is healing for me is...

15 I've learned that...

16 I've changed...

17 The life gifts I've received are...

18 I celebrate by...

19 I commemorate my experience by ...

20 Someone showed me an extra measure of compassion by...

21 I find my internal oasis when...